DEVELOPING
CLINICAL
PROBLEM-SOLVING
SKILLS

HOWARD S. BARROWS, M.D., FRCP(C)

Professor and Chairman, Department of Medical Education;
Professor of Medicine (Neurology);
Associate Dean for Educational Affairs,
Southern Illinois University School of Medicine,
Springfield, Illinois

GARFIELD C. PICKELL, M.D., CCFP, ABFP

Associate Professor of Family Practice,
University of California at Davis;
Medical Director of Ambulatory and Emergency Services,
Scenic General Hospital, Modesto, California;
private practice, Hughson, California

DEVELOPING
CLINICAL
PROBLEM-SOLVING
SKILLS

A Guide to More Effective

Diagnosis and Treatment

Norton Medical Books

W · W · Norton & Company

New York · London

o 5013574

HEALTH SCIENCES

The text of this book is composed in Sabon, with the display set in Friz Qua-
drata. Composition by Arcata Graphics/Kingsport. Manufacturing by Fairfield
Graphics. Book design by Jack Meserole.

First Edition.

ISBN 0-393-71010-6

W.W. Norton & Company, Inc., 500 Fifth Avenue, New York, N.Y. 10110
W.W. Norton & Company, Ltd., 10 Optic Street, London WC1A IPU

1 2 3 4 5 6 7 8 9 0

Contents

creative process. Another crucial step in the clinical-reasoning process now faces you—a step that often separates the novice from the expert. What information is needed to resolve the patient's problem to an appropriate hypothesis? What kinds of questions or examinations can most powerfully or efficiently separate the contending hypotheses? What do you do when the hypotheses do not seem to be verifiable? How can you be certain that other information—not related to your hypotheses, but important to the understanding of your patient's problem—has not been missed?

favor of the patient. There is risk and responsibility in this task. Diagnostic decision-making is one of the great professional challenges in medicine.

Therapeutic Decision-Making   162

11

The therapeutic decision is the whole purpose of your encounter with the patient. Are you able to cure the patient, alleviate his or her symptoms, improve on the natural course of the illness, minimize or avoid complications? Is your treatment worth the cost and potential risk or possible discomfort? Again, choices have to be made sensitive to these benefit/cost factors, the patient's needs, and his or her value system. The choices often have to be made on limited data.

Patient Education   175

12

Your treatment plan is not complete until you have designed an individualized patient education plan. The overall goals of patient education are

1. To ensure compliance. *That is, to provide the patient with enough knowledge and understanding of his problems, of the consequences, and of the expected effects and results of treatment, to enable him to understand and follow instructions and advice, and to recognize when he is satisfactorily performing the responsibilities given to him.*
2. To enable the patient to take appropriate, logical and reasoned actions in dealing with his problems.
3. To enhance healthy behavior. *This involves enabling the patient to modify his behaviors relative to a medical problem.*

Preface

This book is written primarily for medical students, but it will also be of value to residents and practicing physicians. It has two principal objectives. The first is to help you perfect your problem-solving or clinical-reasoning skills so that you can evaluate and treat patients in the most effective and efficient manner. The second is aimed at helping you learn from your work with patient problems in a way that will provide you with a growing, useful body of knowledge that will be more easily recalled and more effectively applied to your clinical work. This is not a book on interview and physical-examination techniques, or a text on the humanistic approach to medical care. Nor is it based on personal introspection and clinical experiences; rather, it has developed through many years of teaching and evaluating the clinical skills of medical students, residents, and practicing physicians and is based on many studies of the expert physician's reasoning process and on studies in cognitive and educational psychology. Over the years we have had the opportunity to study the reasoning processes used by many students, residents, and physicians, using a variety of techniques. A number of the subjects had identified difficulty in clinical work. The problems found in their reasoning have provided much of the impetus for this book.

There are two components of expert clinical problem-solving that need to be considered separately even though they cannot be separated in practice. One is *content,* the rich, extensive knowledge base about medicine that resides in the long-term memory of the expert. The other is *process,* the method of knowledge manipulation the expert uses to apply that knowledge to the patient's problem. In expert performance these components are inexorably intertwined. Both are required; a well-developed reasoning process appropriately bringing accurate knowledge to bear on a problem in the most effective manner.

The concept of metacognition, described in Chapter 2, has allowed the expert's process to be seen as a reflective-thinking skill that is developed through thoughtful practice. This book should help you perfect the *process* of clinical reasoning to best deliver the knowledge that you now have, (and will acquire in the future) to the care of your patients. (Many available textbooks concentrate on the knowledge the clinician must have about diseases and symptoms. Their emphasis is on the *content* aspect of expert clinical performance. Many of these texts are listed in the Selected References. They complement, but do not compete with this book.)

Chapters 13 and 14, especially, tell you how new information about previous patient problems acquired from work and study can be most effectively incorporated into your memory, recalled, and used during your reasoning about a subsequent patient problem. (A review of the chapter summaries in the table of contents will provide you with a quick but more detailed review of the book.)

If you are a medical student, you cannot undertake this book too early, as it will start you on the way to developing professional problem-solving and clinical-reasoning skills. To develop these skills you must practice, analyze, and repractice them until they are automatic. More important, if you associate your medical-school learning with this regimen, your knowledge will be organized for effective recollection in your clinical work.

If you are a resident or practicing physician, this book may help you further develop your clinical-reasoning abilities. The book analyzes in detail the individual steps of the expert physician's clinical-reasoning process. It discusses common problems or bad habits often observed in these steps, and methods for improving performance. This analysis makes you conscious of your own clinical reasoning—normally an unconscious, or automatic process—so that you can perfect each step. The book will help you use your patient experiences to analyze your personal continuing-education needs and to develop self-education skills that will help you to keep your knowledge and skills well honed and up to date.

As mentioned previously, many excellent tests on clinical problem-solving show you how to evaluate and treat a variety of common or important patient problems. This is not such a case-based book. By concentrating on the process of clinical reasoning, as opposed to the specifics of individual cases, this book will help you evaluate *any* patient problem, no matter how rare or complex, and to learn *how* to learn from your patient work.

ACKNOWLEDGMENTS

It would be impossible to give full credit to all of the people who have given help with this book. Charles Engel provided many valuable suggestions that improved the book's ability to communicate with the reader, such as the chapter summaries and marginal notes. Paul Feltovich, Beth Dawson-Saunders, Reed Williams, and Dave Swanson gave advice from their various areas of expertise.

Student feedback is treasured by anyone writing a book for students, and we have many students to thank over a number of years. Among them, Mary Bourland and Jeffrey Frank, once students, but now practicing physicians, deserve special recognition for their detailed critiques and suggestions when they were students.

DEVELOPING
CLINICAL
PROBLEM-SOLVING
SKILLS

1

Introduction

*An overall view of the clinical-reasoning process
as a problem-solving method designed to handle
the problems patients present. The relationship of
this process to medical knowledge is discussed, and
basic terms are defined. The ways in which the
clinician must be prepared for the patient are outlined.*

The emergency-room nurse tells you that Mr.
Hawkins, a 54-year-old who has never been in
before, is complaining of chest pain. When you
walk in, a mildly obese man sits on the examining
table. He is bent forward, bearing his weight on
hands that grasp the edge of the table. He does
not seem to be in distress. His wife is with him,
and she seems anxious. After you introduce yourself, Mr. Hawkins says, "I have this persistent pain
in my chest that won't go away. It feels like indigestion."

What is your responsibility here? What are you
going to do? Is this a heart problem, or is it something else? Are you going to have to act quickly,
even initiate some treatment, or can you take your
time?

You may not have time to ask a lot of questions—What are the best questions to ask? Should you do a complete physical examination, or just concentrate on a few important steps? What are the important ones?

THE CHALLENGE OF THE PATIENT'S PROBLEM

The information available at the outset of a patient encounter is usually insufficient to arrive at any kind of diagnostic conclusion. Before the patient's problem can be defined well enough to allow for treatment decisions, no matter how urgent treatment may be, more information is needed. In addition, there is no one correct or prescribed way to get this information for a particular patient's problem. Give the same patient problem to ten expert clinicians and you will get ten different approaches to obtaining more information, each using somewhat different questions and requiring different physical-examination procedures in different sequences. Nevertheless, the approaches will usually provide the same diagnostic conclusions, each based on different clusters of facts about the patient.

As new information is discovered in the interview and examination, the picture presented by the patient at the outset may change and, not infrequently will become quite a different problem than suspected. A physical complaint, such as chest pain, could turn out to be a psychological problem, such as chronic stress-induced anxiety. Conversely, a patient presenting with a history very typical of depression may eventually be found to have pancreatic or colonic carcinoma, or a brain tumor. Occasionally, the person presenting to the clinician is found not to be the patient at all, but to be troubled with symptoms induced by the psychiatric problems of another family member.

Ambiguities and conflicting or inadequate information are the rule in medicine. You can never be sure that you have really solved a patient problem, you can only be confident of approaching a solution.

These qualities—the inadequate information at the outset, the lack of definite guidelines for working up the problem, the mutability of the problem, and the lack of assurance that the problem has been solved—are not unique to patient problems. They are characteristic of all *ill-structured problems*, which are encountered in most professions. They determine the reasoning processes that have to be employed to evaluate and treat patient problems. If information is insufficient to define or diagnose at the outset, then a variety of possible diagnoses or *hypotheses* suggested by the available information have to be considered to determine what further information is needed. An *inquiry strategy*, guided by these hypotheses, has to be designed to obtain the appropriate facts. There is little point in asking any question that comes to mind. Hypotheses serve as a guide to the kinds of facts that are needed. As the inquiry takes place, the new information obtained from the patient is analyzed. The data that seem significant in the light of the suggested hypotheses has to be added or *synthesized* to the problem in order to progressively define the problem. Since you will rarely find all the information you need to make a definitive diagnosis, you will usually have to make a

The strategies necessary to cope with ill-structured problems dictate the nature of the clinical-reasoning process.

diagnostic decision on the basis of probability. The thinking stages that are required to cope with the patient's ill-structured problem are exactly those seen in studies of the clinical-reasoning process of the physician.

THE CLINICAL-REASONING PROCESS

Over the last few years, findings from a variety of formal studies of the physician have provided a consistent model of the clinician's problem-solving process (see Selected References). A model developed from these studies will be used to help you develop effective professional skills to evaluate and care for your patients. It is the same model that logic would design to cope with any ill-structured problem.

The detective, scientist, mechanic, and physician all employ professional deductive-reasoning skills, using multiple hypotheses.

This model resembles the approach of a detective faced with a crime, a scientist confronted with an unexplained phenomenon, or a mechanic confronted with a malfunctioning piece of equipment. In each of these situations, a problem is presented of which a cause is not immediately apparent, and a number of different causes or hypotheses are entertained. The information necessary to decide which causes are correct requires a search for further information, interrogation of witnesses, or a search for clues by the detective; observation and experimentation by the scientist; a check into various mechanical systems by the mechanic; and interview and examination of the patient by the physician.

The possible places in which the detective could search for further clues are infinite. The measurements, studies, and analyses the scientist could carry out are endless. A mechanic could take apart the entire machine and check every part. In the same manner, the physician could ask a thousand questions, perform an endless physical examination, and order a hundred tests. None of these professionals do this. They could waste a good deal of time, effort, and money before finding information relevant to resolving the problem. Instead, they use several causes (or hypotheses) suggested by the problem to determine exactly what information they need to deduce a most likely hypothesis.

The multiple-hypothetics—deductive method contains what would be an otherwise infinite search.

All of these professionals use multiple hypotheses generated early in the problem encounter to guide their inquiry. As they inquire—the detective after clues, the scientist after relevant data, the mechanic after malfunctions, and the physician after symptoms and signs—they collect an increasingly large amount of information. In order to retain this information effectively in their search for the most likely hypothesis, all these professionals assemble or synthesize the data they feel are important into an evolving mental image of the problem. At some point they decide which of their hypotheses match this evolving picture most closely. Often there is a poor match, and new hypotheses have to be generated to guide further inquiry until a close enough match is found to allow for a decision as to the cause of the crime, natural phenomenon, malfunctioning car, or patient's problem.

Other stages in the process are synthesizing the significant data and making decisions.

This is the problem-solving, decision-making process. Subsequent chapters will elaborate on specific stages of the process as they apply to the

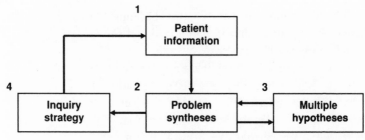

FIGURE 1. The basic structure of the clinical-reasoning process: (1) initial patient information is (2) synthesized into the patient problem. (3) The clinician creates hypotheses about the possible causes for this problem, which serve as a guide for (4) the inquiry strategy.

Stages of the physician's clinical-reasoning process: hypothesis generation, inquiry strategy, data analysis, problem synthesis, diagnostic and treatment decision-making.

physician: (1) hypothesis generation, (2) inquiry strategy, (3) data analysis, (4) problem synthesis, (5) diagnostic and treatment decision-making. Figure 1 shows the relationship of these stages to one another. This basic flow chart will grow with subsequent figures in each chapter, illustrating how each stage fits into the overall process.

This is the way the good physician thinks, whether consciously or not. This problem-solving behavior is often performed so quickly, so reflexively, that the skilled problem-solver is unaware of the process. On introspection, many physicians think they use only *intuition* to arrive at a diagnosis. Others feel that they gather all the necessary data first and then decide on a diagnosis. Despite these opinions, carefully performed studies show that most physicians employ the multiple-staged method described above, even in situations where the diagnosis may seem obvious.

This multiple-hypothesis, guided-inquiry, problem-synthesis, and decision behavior best exemplifies the physician's first contact with a patient.

Follow-up examinations and routine checkups also employ this process, but in a modified and sometimes fragmented form.

Depending on your level of training in medicine and the amount of experience you have had with patients, you might feel that you don't have enough knowledge to come up with the appropriate hypotheses in a particular case. That may not really be true. In the case of Mr. Hawkins (introduced at the beginning of the chapter), if you ask yourself what could be the possible causes for chest pain in a 54-year-old man—knowing all the structures that are contained in the chest and recalling anything you have heard, seen, or experienced about chest pain—you can come up with a number of ideas that could guide your questions. Don't worry about that now; you will confront Mr. Hawkins again in most of the following chapters, as we consider each step in the clinician's reasoning process and how it should be practiced and developed. However, it is important to understand at the outset the relationship between the clinician's reasoning process and the amount of knowledge the physician has.

THE RELATIONSHIP OF KNOWLEDGE TO CLINICAL REASONING

Many have the erroneous idea that the general form of the physician's clinical-reasoning process varies substantially with different problems and with different medical specialties. This error occurs

The complex relationship between reasoning skills (process) and available knowledge (content) must be understood.

when the scientific method as a *process* is not considered separately from the factual knowledge that the clinician may have acquired.

If a clinician has had extensive experience with certain patient problems, he will easily recall the most effective hypotheses or diagnoses when confronted by that problem. The clinician also will recall the best inquiry strategy to use with that problem—which questions to ask and which examinations to perform—to deduce the correct diagnosis quickly. That inquiry strategy employs those few questions, examinations, and tests that experience has repeatedly shown to discriminate most accurately and efficiently between the diagnostic hypotheses. Also, because of that experience, the clinician will also note certain small cues or variations in the patient's complaint or appearance that will suggest more likely diagnoses. Thus the experienced clinician's evaluation often is more effective and rapid than that of an uninitiated or less experienced clinician. For example, a primary-care physician faced with a short-of-breath child may come up with a wide range of general hypotheses. After many questions, the physician refines these hypotheses, making them more specific. Eventually a totally new set of hypotheses may be required. An extensive examination and a number of laboratory tests may be needed to get enough information for a decision. By contrast, an experienced pediatric cardiologist who has worked with this kind of problem many times can pick up many subtle cues from the patient's age, appearance, and description of the shortness of breath, and quickly generate one or two sophisticated hypotheses. The specialist may ask only a few questions, put a stethoscope to the child's chest, hear what would be to most physicians a subtle sound, and make the correct diagnosis. The two physicians may seem to have used different processes. Yet they both derived hypotheses and acquired data to confirm or deny these hypotheses, and then came to a diagnostic decision. The cardiologist's particular memory files, related to a particular patient population with characteristic diagnostic probabilities, offered valuable shortcuts: process (clinical reasoning) and content (clinical knowledge) worked together. With rich, sophisticated content the process may be quick and incisive. (However, with puzzling, complex problems, for which little helpful information can be recalled, the process may be extended and circular even in the specialist's hands.)

Hematologists may not emphasize extensive histories or physical examinations. Instead the nature of their specialty calls them to depend upon an array of laboratory studies. Symptoms and signs may not be helpful in distinguishing different hematologic conditions. The reasoning of these clinicians is no different; only their data source is different. They get more valuable data to sort out their hypotheses from laboratory tests. They still generate hypotheses, but they inquire principally through laboratory studies to resolve these hypotheses.

No one can apply the clinical scientific method to patients' problems effectively without the knowledge to generate appropriate hypotheses. Knowledge is needed to devise questions or examinations to rule hypotheses in or out, and to decide eventually on the correct hypothesis and treatment. As you work with more and more patient problems and you acquire more knowledge, your memory becomes enriched with numerous associations that

The fundamental mental process is the same, whether a clinician takes shortcuts with a familiar problem or performs an extensive history and physical with an unfamiliar problem.

will come to mind when you face a new patient problem. For certain recurring problems you will develop routines that get to the heart of the matter quickly.

For example, even before seeing a patient with the very common complaint of "sore throat," the clinician may have essentially decided on a treatment plan. He will likely have developed a very brief, routine, and systematic interview and examination for this complaint, designed to confirm the most probable hypothesis—upper respiratory infection (URI) (bacterial or viral)—and to rule out more significant or unusual conditions for which there is specific treatment or which require further investigation. Specific questions and examinations would be directed toward ruling out hypotheses such as

- otitis media (red tympanic membrane)
- purulent sinusitis (purulent nasal discharge and tender maxillary and frontal sinuses)
- acute tonsillitis (very large acutely inflamed tonsils)
- lower respiratory infection, including pneumonia (production of purulent sputum, shortness of breath, rigors and chills and pleuritic chest pain, adventitious sounds on auscultation)
- asthma (wheezing on auscultation)

In special circumstances, questions and examination might be directed toward unusual problems endemic to certain times and places, such as oral candidiasis, diphtheria, chemical inhalation, or gonococcal pharyngitis. Complex as this sounds, it is generally accomplished in less than a minute. The clinician then proceeds with the almost predetermined treatment plan [which is usually the same for either viral or bacterial URI since it is impossible to tell the difference until culture results are available (some clinicians rely on a streptococcal enzyme test)].

If you work and study in a specialty, you will develop sophisticated facts and strategies for specialty-related problems. Chapters 13 and 14 will help you incorporate your learning to support your clinical-reasoning process effectively.

Throughout our professional lives we encounter patient problems for which our knowledge and experience are inadequate. You must prepare for these baffling cases by developing effective and secure clinical-reasoning strategies to carry you as far as your knowledge will allow. Expect these problems to occur less and less frequently as you go through undergraduate, postgraduate, and practice experiences. However, when the situation occurs, good clinical-reasoning skills using well-thought-out hypotheses based on what you do know, the use of an inquiry strategy based on what information you do have, and a synthesis of the problem that is as accurate as possible will carry you very far in working with such a patient problem. In addition, if you can develop a well-tuned awareness of your limitations, and if you identify the kinds of knowledge you need to acquire to make a better diagnostic evaluation and to undertake a better plan of treatment with that patient, and then return to the patient having learned that information, your patient will have profited and so will you. This method of problem-based, self-directed learning—a powerful and well-established learning method—is emphasized throughout this

Good reasoning skills will carry you a long way even if you're short on needed facts.

The "knowledge-bound" student or physician.

book. A secure and professional process of clinical reasoning and an adequate knowledge base are both essential and relate closely to each other.

The possession of an encyclopedic memory of facts and concepts in basic and clinical science certainly will not ensure effective evaluation of your patient's problem. You have to know how to apply that information to the problem in the evaluation and treatment of your patient. There are many "knowledge-bound" students and physicians, who can pass oral or written examinations well and give brilliant discussions, but who are incapable of caring for patients efficiently or properly. Their clinical-reasoning process is defective or rudimentary.

The same relationship between your knowledge and your reasoning skills can be seen when you learn a new game, or learn how to operate a computer. In the beginning you go through laborious operations and mental deliberations. After experience and knowledge are acquired, playing the game or operating the equipment becomes a nearly automatic behavior in almost any circumstance. Remember, however, that the basic reasoning process is always present, and that it needs to be performed well.

This book is designed to help you develop the reasoning skills you need to work effectively with your patients. It will also give you techniques to build your clinical knowledge from patient experiences in ways that will reinforce your reasoning.

Early patient experiences allow for practice, and enhance medical-school learning.

Early development of these clinical-reasoning skills will allow medical students to make the most of clinical opportunities during their undergraduate education. In their work with patients, medical students and physicians alike must always be aware of how well they are performing at every stage, and where they need to improve upon their performance.

TERMS AND DEFINITIONS

Some definitions follow for terms that will be used throughout this book. You may find some of these definitions to be somewhat idiosyncratic. However, they reflect usage within the book and should be kept in mind.

PATIENT: A person with a known or suspected health problem who has entered a professional relationship with a physician for reasons related to that problem.

SETTING: The place in which the patient-clinician encounter occurs (such as an office, emergency room, primary-care clinic, specialty clinic, or hospital ward). Setting is important, as it implies a different goal for the physician and different expectations by the patient.

EVALUATION: Questions, examinations, and tests and other diagnostic procedures are all *actions* used in the inquiry by the clinician to evaluate the patient's problem.

TREATMENT/MANAGEMENT: Actions used to help the patient with his or her problem. They include writing prescriptions; giving injections or instrumentations (lumbar puncture, intubation, intravenous infusions); performing surgery; providing counseling or education; arranging for admission to a hospital; making referrals; prescribing physical therapy; and so on.

CLINICIAN: The person encountering the patient in a professional relationship, who evaluates the problem and provides treatment. The clinician can be a medical student, resident, or physician, or a nurse or nursing student.

DIAGNOSIS: Usually this term implies a formal statement of the clinician's decision as to the most likely cause of the patient's problem. Many modifying terms are used.

probable diagnosis

working diagnosis

tentative diagnosis

diagnostic impression (*or just* impression)

Each denotes the best guess of the moment in the clinician's ongoing evaluation of the patient's problem. Each is subject to change on the basis of new or subsequent information. *Hypothesis* (discussed below) is a more general term that encompasses all of the above terms.

FINAL DIAGNOSIS: This term implies that there is no question left as to the correctness of the diagnosis.

DIFFERENTIAL DIAGNOSIS: A list of alternative diagnoses still to be considered at the end of the inquiry. These are hypotheses that could not be eliminated during the investigation of the patient's problem.

It is unfortunate that *diagnosis* usually suggests a label that is specific, or related to specific organ system diseases. The diagnostic decision made at the end of the patient encounter must be no more specific than the data obtained during the investigation of the patient will allow. Very effective practicing clinicians frequently conclude their investigation of patients with such general diagnoses as "a liver disorder" or "something wrong with the cervical spinal cord" or similar broad strokes of the diagnostic brush when the information available is insufficient to draw a more specific diagnosis. This prevents the physician from coming to conclusions that are too refined and suggests the need for more investigation through tests or diagnostic procedures.

Diagnostic decisions *must* include psychological, social, ethical, and economic factors. The clinician must label *all* problems affecting the patient's health so that the management of each is undertaken.

HYPOTHESIS: Hypotheses can be descriptions of

disease processes

pathological processes

clinical entities

clinical syndromes

physiological derangements

etiological processes

affected organs or tissues

psychological processes

social or economic factors

or whatever labels that best explain the possible causes for the patient's problem. Initial hypotheses are working guides in clinical reasoning and are subject to change and refinement. At the end of the patient encounter, the clinician still has working hypotheses subject to verification or change as tests are ordered and the patient is followed. It is best to think of diagnoses as working hypotheses. (This concept is elaborated further in Chapter 3.)

CLINICAL PROBLEM-SOLVING/THE CLINICAL SCIENTIFIC METHOD/CLINICAL REASONING: Terms used interchangeably to refer to the problem-solving process clinicians employ with patient problems.

PRELIMINARIES

Before any patient encounter, you should consider a number of items that have a direct bearing on the success of the encounter, items that are often either tacitly assumed or not thought about at all.

The Implicit Contract

A tacit contract, influenced by the setting, always exists between patient and clinician.

The professional service implied by the setting in which you encounter the patient provides an implicit contract. The setting creates certain expectations in the mind of the patient. It also implies a specific set of goals for the clinician. An emergency-room encounter usually implies a quick decision about either hospitalization, immediate treatment actions, or referral for care elsewhere. It is not the place for a lengthy evaluation of complex or chronic medical or psychosocial complaints. The emergency-room contact is usually a one-time-only affair with no follow-up. The specialty or outpatient clinic implies a careful investigation into the health problems related to that specialty. It also implies extensive or elaborate laboratory tests and other diagnostic procedures, as well as treatments. Primary-care outpatient settings (as in family practice, general practice, or pediatrics) usually imply brief visits to evaluate and treat minor or common complaints. It may also imply continuing care, with referral to other health specialists for more complex or exotic problems. An inpatient encounter on a hospital ward or in a room usually implies extensive investigations or treatments that are impossible or inconvenient to perform outside the hospital. It can imply a serious illness. In this setting the patient has invariably seen a clinician who has arranged for the admission and made decisions as to what should occur during hospitalization. The same settings in different parts of the country or in different communities may have varied implications. You should consider what the contract is for the particular setting in which you encounter the patient.

You should determine the tacit or implied services that your patient expects from you. They may be different than you might assume. Any difference in assumed contract between the patient and yourself leads to problems in both communications and compliance. For example, it is common for patients who come to a specialty clinic to assume that their complaint will be correctly diagnosed and they will be given appropriate treatment. This is often suggested by the referring physician. The patient may come to a primary-care setting with a conviction as to what is wrong and which treatments he should receive, yet never verbalize that expectation. You may find to your surprise that your patient didn't even want to come, but did so only at the insistence of a spouse, employer,

The clinician's and the patient's tacit assumptions may not match.

teacher, or referring physician. Beware of tacit expectations both on *your* part and the *patient's*. Decide which objectives are appropriate to the setting, and discuss them with the patient. Your objectives will determine the time you are going to spend with the patient: a short time for triage in a emergency-room setting, a longer time for a problem in a primary-care setting, and a longer, more detailed investigation in a specialty setting. You will look for life-threatening problems in the emergency room, surgically treatable problems in the surgery clinic, common medical or psychological problems in primary care, and sophisticated specific organ problems in specialty areas.

However, you must *always* be concerned about *all* the problems the patient may have in *any* setting, and make certain that they are appropriately cared for by someone. Awareness of the contract affects your inquiry strategy and decision-making process.

In all settings the clinician must be certain to recognize all the patient's potential problems, even if some are to be addressed at another time or by someone else.

The Clinician's Role

What is your role in the patient encounter? As either a medical student or resident, this is an important decision for you to make. Is it your responsibility to evaluate and care for the patient, or are you an intermediary whose job it is to gather the facts and pass them on to someone else? In both instances you will have to be a problem-solver, but in the latter you will have the burden of communicating the patient's picture accurately and free of interpretive biases, and being thorough enough in the details of your investigation that the person to whom you present the problem gets an accurate picture. This is a common situation for medical students. As students gain more experience and the physician to whom they present the patient problem gains confidence in their skills, they are usually allowed increasing responsibility in decision-making. If you don't know your role, find out.

Attitudes, Time Constraints, Pressures

Review your commitment to the patient in your encounter. If you have many pressures on you, or if you are uncomfortable about the setting or the patient, you may not be prepared to give proper service.

Unrecognized factors can adversely affect the quality and the success of the clinician-patient encounter.

Even though you are an intelligent, dedicated person you possibly could dislike psychiatric patients, neurological patients, geriatric patients, or others. Look carefully at yourself. If you can discover such inherent prejudicial attitudes, awareness will help you compensate. However, you should look into the possible reasons for your attitudes—which we all have—and see if you can change the attitudes. If not, they might indicate the kinds of practice you should avoid in your career.

You may have many patients waiting outside in the clinic, problems on the ward, or other pressures. These pressures may adversely affect your commitment to the patient and to the careful analysis of the patient's problems that unfold in the encounter. You might unconsciously take shortcuts; look for the easier, more obvious explanations for the patient's problem; take less time to inquire about complexities; pick easy, less involved, but perhaps inappropriate therapies; or order a whole array of unnecessary tests as a substitute for a careful history and physical examination.

It is not fair to any patient for a clinician's pressures or attitudes to hamper the quality of their care.

If your commitment is really not as it should be, take stock of the situation and *do something positive:*

recognize what is going on and become committed to the patient; or

arrange for the patient to be seen by someone else; or

arrange for your other burdens to be cared for by others, or deferred.

HOW TO USE THIS BOOK

To make the most of the method presented in this book you must practice. To do this you need to have patient problems available. Written case histories are not adequate; since all the needed information about the patient is provided, you cannot practice the initial stages of the clinical-reasoning process. However, if you team up with someone, an extensive case history can be useful. Work with real patients, simulated patients, or specially designed simulation formats (available in print and on computer software). Some available patient simulations are listed in the Selected References. Your access to appropriate patient problems that feature the particular subjects you are studying in medical school greatly enhance the value of this book. If you are in the clinical-clerkship period or beyond, you have access to patients. However, if you are in the first couple of years of medical school and there are no simulations or patients available, you must either obtain your own problem simulations or find a clinician you can work with during off

Find a way to experience pertinent contact from the very beginning of medical school.

hours. Chapter 12 describes how you can set up your clinical experiences to develop your clinical-reasoning skills, and to help you better understand and retain what you are learning in medical school.

2

Intuition and Metacognition

What is called intuition in diagnosis can be attributed to the recollection of forgotten facts, to automatic thinking, or to the unconscious processing of an apparently insoluble problem. Metacognition refers to the processes of deliberation and reflection during problem-solving. It is the hallmark of the expert clinician.

INTUITION, THE UNEXPECTED SOLUTION

The term *intuition* tends to cover a variety of mental activities. In medicine it is often used to label a clinician's decision about correct diagnosis or treatment when sufficient objective evidence or clear-cut reasons for that decision are not available, and is described as characteristic of the experienced clinician. The usual implication is that there was no deliberation on the part of the clinician, who just unerringly "knew" the right choices by virtue of expertise or prior experiences. An additional and unfortunate implication is that intuition must be an "art" that cannot be taught—something that is magically acquired only through experience. Actually, you can develop this power of intuition early on, by the way you learn and apply new information. Acquiring new information while you are struggling with a problem and applying that information to the problem will better ensure future recall. This book provides you with a learning approach that will facilitate effective, efficient, and fast clinical-reasoning skills—the skills behind intuition.

In some instances, intuition represents the recall of previously learned but seemingly forgotten facts from deep within long-term memory. In medical practice this often results when a particular complex of symptoms or signs in a patient triggers memory of facts associated with prior patient problems.

Intuition also may represent rapid, automatic thinking. Experience with certain types of patient problems engenders familiarity with relevant diagnostic ideas, or hypotheses, and the specific questions, physical-examination items, and laboratory tests that will be called for. They pop into mind automatically as if with no effort. It is like driving a car; it is done so often that the many decisions and manipulations necessary to deal with the problems that appear on the way (traffic, weather, road conditions, pedestrians) all become so ingrained that they are performed quickly and without much conscious thought. However, much unconscious, rapid problem-solving is going on. If after arriving at a familiar location a driver were asked to recall the thought processes and actions involved in getting there, he would not be able to recall them

Intuition may involve rapid, automatic thinking, or the recollection of forgotten facts. It can be developed.

and would feel that he "just drove there"—that no particular thought was involved. This behavior occurs frequently with expert clinicians. They will zero in on just the right questions and without apparent deliberation come to an almost magical diagnostic conclusion—and not be able to describe why they did what they did. This is not so magical. You too will show these behaviors with problems that recur frequently. In some instances this automatic behavior may blind the clinician to subtle variations or cues in the problem that need to be noticed and consciously thought about as they could point to an unanticipated diagnosis or complication. This needed conscious thought is referred to in the next section.

Intuition is that "Eureka!" that strikes you later out of a clear blue sky: the voice of your unconscious.

As a term, *intuition* is probably best reserved for the sudden, unexpected solution to a patient problem that comes to mind after giving the matter considerable deliberation with no avail. There seems to be no way to put the problem together or decide what to do upon a conscious review of the available evidence. This unexpected solution may occur some time after the problem has been puzzled over, during what seems to be intellectually neutral activity, when the mind wanders with no particular agenda—such as when in bed, while driving, in the shower, and so on. It is as if the unconscious mind had been searching through an abandoned leg of a mine and suddenly hit pay dirt. "Eureka," the solution appears in the conscious mind. This intuition is valuable and has to be used with imponderables. It can often be counted upon if you consciously and carefully review your difficult patient problem in every way you can, backwards and forwards, and then "put it on the back burner" for a while, tackling other tasks and letting the unconscious mind work.

Intuitive ideas and decisions also tend to appear under emergency conditions when answers to a difficult or perplexing problem have to be found. Feeling that it is not scientific to trust intuition, many people are not sensitive to their intuitions. Try trusting your intuition when your back is against the wall and you cannot, despite all rational conscious effort, come to a decision when you really must.

Intuition is a useful skill, which you should develop.

METACOGNITION, HALLMARK OF THE PROFESSIONAL

Metacognition refers to the voluntary, conscious, and self-monitoring act of thinking. It is the opposite of impulsive reflex thinking. It entails putting conscious effort into thinking. Such words as *pondering, deliberating, cogitating,* or *reflecting* describe metacognition. Note that a self-monitoring function is also implied in this term. Besides pondering or reflecting over a perplexing situation, the clinician should be asking himself how well he is doing in thinking through the problem: does he need help, advice, more information? In *The Reflective Practitioner* Donald Schön calls these metacognitive skills of professionals *reflection-in-action.*

Metacognition involves deliberation, reflection, as well as the monitoring of one's own thinking.

This book is aimed at helping you develop effective metacognitive skills to monitor your clinical-reasoning process and your continued learning. Each chapter addresses a component of the clinical-

The development of metacognitive skills in clinical reasoning and self-education is vital.

reasoning process and describes the kinds of questions you should be asking yourself in monitoring your own thinking as you work with patient problems. Whenever something does not seem right—the symptoms or signs are not typical, something the patient says cannot be readily understood, the laboratory findings do not make sense, or whatever—you must stop, review, and deliberate. In truth, if metacognition were generally better understood, the most accurate title for this book would be *Developing the Metacognitive Skills Necessary for Continued, Successful Practice in Medicine.*

3

Forming the Initial
Concept

When you first see your patient, an initial, general question or two will usually encourage the patient to describe his or her symptoms or concerns. As the patient talks, you may notice the patient's appearance, facial expression, posture, movements, dress and voice. In addition, you may have in your possession prior medical records or referral notes about your patient. From this wealth of initially available information you must pick out the facts or observations that seem most important. With this information the clinician almost automatically decides whether there is a problem and what kind of problem it might be. This is the initial concept.

THE START OF THE PATIENT
ENCOUNTER

At the beginning of the patient encounter—when you first see the patient and begin to interact—a limited amount of data is already available to start your clinical-reasoning process:

1. the patient's opening complaints, comments, and responses to your initial questions
2. the patient's appearance, age, sex, physiognomy, dress and posture
3. the patient's movements and speech characteristics such as animation, clarity, rise and fall of the voice
4. appearance and manner of people with the patient (spouse, parent, friend, guardian, nurse)

These initially available data stimulate the clinician to form an initial concept about the nature of the problem he is about to tackle.

MR. HAWKINS*

You are a primary-care clinician working in an emergency room. You are going to see Mr. Bill Hawkins, who is complaining of chest pain. The initial information, presented to you by the nurse on the emergency-room data sheet before you see the patient, is as follows:

Mr. Hawkins is a 54-year-old man with chest pain. He has never been here before.

You note that his vital signs, as recorded, are normal.

As you enter the room you see that Mr. Hawkins appears to be about his stated age of 54. He is mildly obese, casually dressed, and appears to be sweating although the room and outside temperatures are cool. He is not

* Mr. Hawkins was introduced in Chapter 1. You will be working with him throughout the book.

otherwise in obvious distress. He is sitting on the examining table, bent forward and bearing his weight on his hands, which are grasping the edge of the table. His speech is clear and slightly hurried, with an anxious tone. He is accompanied by his wife, who appears anxious.

After you introduce yourself, Mr. Hawkins says, "I have this persistent pain in my chest that won't go away. It feels like indigestion."

You note brown stains on Mr. Hawkins's right second and third fingers, and an odor characteristic of distilled spirits.

What is your *initial concept* of this patient? Write it on a piece of paper. You should always have a note pad with you in clinical work to record your ideas, data you want to remember, and questions to be answered.

The Presenting Complaint

From the initially available data experienced clinicians automatically perceive those that may seem unusual and will look for others that may be significant in the light of the patient's reason for coming. For example, if the patient complains of shortness of breath, the clinician may look for ankle swelling, increased rate of breathing, and an altered pattern and distention of neck veins, because shortness of breath is a common symptom for cardiac failure and these observations would reinforce that possibility. Such observations would constitute a visual inquiry in response to the clinician's entertained hypothesis of congestive heart failure.

The initial concept is derived from observations deliberately sought and noted.

Other Factors Affecting the Initial Concept

If there is nothing unusual about the patient's appearance or manner of movement, the clinician's initial concept of the patient's problem may indeed *be* the patient's presenting complaint. For example, if a normal-appearing young woman complains of constant pain in the upper abdomen over the last few weeks, the clinician's initial concept more than likely will be simply "a young woman with constant upper abdominal pain of a few weeks duration." However, if this woman presents with downcast eyes, a quiet voice, a face with little expression, little animation in body movement, and complains of upper abdominal pain, the clinician initial concept may well be, "a depressed-appearing young woman with constant upper abdominal pain for the last few weeks." These two initial concepts are quite different and each would direct the clinician's initial diagnostic hypotheses and inquiry in quite different directions, the latter involving more emphasis on psychosocial and psychiatric areas.

The initial concept may be more than the patient's complaint.

Think of any initial complaint a patient may offer. Picture the patient with that complaint in your mind's eye, and state your initial concept. Now picture that patient

1. appearing with slurred speech
2. appearing with agitated behavior and sitting on the edge of the chair
3. appearing with a hostile and exasperated-appearing spouse
4. appearing with eyes that do not look at you but furtively glance about the room
5. making the additional comment, "I was liter-

ally forced to come here as I don't think there is really anything wrong with me."

Note how your initial concept changed with each of the additional observations. Sometimes it will be apparent from the patient's manner that the complaint is not really the important problem, but only an excuse for coming to see the clinician. A worried expression may indicate that there are concerns beyond the facts expressed.

The initial concept may be different from the patient's complaint.

Mr. Hawkins

The clinician's initial concept of Mr. Hawkins, described a few pages ago, is:

A middle-aged, moderately obese, probably sedentary male who drinks and smokes, with new onset of chest pain that seems visceral.*

The clinician has noticed, almost unconsciously, that Mr. Hawkins's employment is recorded on the data sheet as "postal clerk," and that his physiognomy suggests inactivity, leading to the *tentative* assumption that Mr. Hawkins is sedentary (an assumption to be confirmed by questions). The clinician has also noted, again, almost unconsciously, a faint smell of metabolic products of alcoholic drink in the room, that Mr. Hawkins's grey mustache is stained brown along the edge of his lip, and that there are tobacco stains between the second and third fingers of his right hand.

* *Visceral* implies that the pain originates from dysfunctions in an organ within the body cavity as opposed to the chest wall.

The clinician's other tentative assumption is that the pain is visceral. This assumption (also to be tested by history and physical) is based on a sensed similarity between this patient and previous patients with visceral chest pain, on observations that Mr. Hawkins is sweating (an autonomic response to deep visceral pain), that he seems to be in some distress from the pain, that both he and his wife appear very concerned, and that he has some of the apparent risk factors associated with a variety of internal-organ diseases (alcohol consumption, smoking, and obesity).

Additional Sources of Initial Information

There may be additional initial information about the patient available to you before or during the encounter, such as

prior health records

a referral letter

telephone comments or prior comments from spouse, parents, or other relatives; teachers or other school officials; a social worker or nurse; a receptionist; or any person with knowledge of the patient.

Your initial concept should include any valuable data you find from these sources added to the initial data you get from the patient. Be careful that these sources do not bias you by any opinions expressed in such phrases as "an awkward child," "unable to cope," "hypochondriac," and so on.

Prior health records or referral letters provide prior diagnoses or treatments to add to your initial concept. The referral letter may help you determine the nature of your implicit contract with the patient (see Chapter 1 for a discussion of the implicit contract). You may wish to return to these records later as a source for more detailed data in your ongoing evaluation of the patient.

PERCEPTION IN THE PATIENT ENCOUNTER

The experienced clinician pulls together the initially important data and observations from the information available during the early moments of the encounter and assembles them into an initial concept, almost immediately and almost automatically. (These rapid, automatic steps are shown in Figure 2.) He may not always be conscious of what is going on, however, the formation of the initial concept is not a passive process. You only see what you *look* at—what is in focus in the center of your vision. Try looking at one word in the center of this page and notice how few of the others can be read without moving your eyes. Recordings of eye movements show that when a subject looks at a face or a picture, his gaze darts from key point to key point. Memory assembles all the images from each key point into a concept, or mental image, of the object being viewed. To fully see the patient, you have to move your eyes around so that the many vital impressions each fall on the maculae of your retinae. You have to look at the patient carefully to really see him.

If you don't look for it, you won't see it. If you don't listen or sniff for it, you won't hear or smell it.

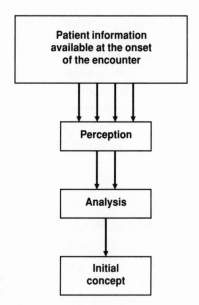

FIGURE 2. The information perceived at the beginning of the encounter is analyzed and assembled into an initial concept.

The Importance of Details

If you look directly at something, you may not notice some details. Few people can recall with confidence the details of a penny, despite how often they may have looked at pennies over the many years of their life. It is rarely important to know those details in order to recognize and use the coin, so you never look at these details. But you have to look at details with your patient.

So it is with listening as well. You may have heard a symphony many times, but until some comment is made about the oboe's part, for example, you may never have noticed that part before.

Similarly, when you are listening to a patient's heart sounds, an S_3 or S_4 is often so inconspicuous (due to its softness and its integration into the rhythms of the louder sounds) that you will not hear it unless—owing to the nature of the patient's problem or history—you are listening specifically for it.

Smells can be quite subtle and can affect our thinking without our being aware of it. We may process smells unconsciously and remain unconscious of their effect on our conclusions. Many disease states have characteristic smells, but the recognition of these smells must be cultivated. Infections such as *Pseudomonas* and *Staphylococcus aureus* have characteristic smells. An alcoholic's breath has a characteristic "hangover" smell, and a chronic alcoholic a characteristic body odor. Ketosis, urinary incontinence, and liver failure have more obtrusive smells.

Recall that Mr. Hawkins's clinician looked for risk factors besides obesity in a man with visceral chest pain—she also smelled for them.

Look at everything that could be significant in the patient's appearance: face, body, hands, etc. Listen, even smell, consciously.

THE HAZARD OF BIAS

Even if you do pick out cues from the patient's conversation or appearance, you may often interpret their significance in light of your past experience, beliefs, assumptions, and prejudices. These biasing factors, added to expectations based on your prior experience with patients, not only determine what information is perceived but how the information is interpreted. For example, a tired-appearing housewife may be assessed as "neurotic." A straight-backed, fussily-dressed patient with rimless glasses may be stereotyped as rigid or judgmental. These biases are often unconscious

Don't color the patient with your biases or prejudices.

and can markedly weaken the effectiveness and objectivity of your evaluation of the patient.

In the following example, the clinician is working in a walk-in clinic, where his function is to quickly assess and manage straightforward problems and to triage more complicated problems. The objective, or contract, for complicated problems in such a setting is to assess their severity and urgency, and arrange appropriate evaluation and follow up, either by himself or by referral. Time with each patient is very limited, and therefore the management objectives are limited to providing treatment for the patient's immediate needs and initiating arrangements for appropriate longer-term evaluation and treatment.

EXAMPLE

Mr. M., a 54-year-old Saudi Arabian Bedouin immigrant, presented—accompanied by his wife—complaining of bilateral ankle pain associated with activity, gradually increasing over the past six months. Mr. M. does not yet speak English; his wife translates. He has been in the United States for six years and is employed in a lumber warehouse, where he is on his feet most of the working day.

The clinician's initial observations include an awareness of Mr. M.'s work clothes, and Mrs. M.'s traditional-appearing Eastern clothing. Mr. M. appears quite shy and he walks rather clumsily—as if he is not quite sure where his feet are—although he does not appear to be in much discomfort.

While talking to the patient through his wife, the clinician begins a screening exam and notes that Mr. M. has lax ankle joints without signs of inflammation and without significant deformity. He has significant loss of light-touch, pin-prick, and vibration sense throughout his feet. He has normal muscle contours and muscle strength in his legs and feet, and has good vascular supply to his feet.

Pathophysiologically, the clinician suspects that the joint problem and resulting pain are due to relative "overuse" and wear secondary to underlying sensory loss with a related loss of protective neural reflexes. That is, pathophysiologically he appears to have a trophic osteoarthritis secondary to an underlying peripheral neuropathy.

His concept of the patient becomes:

> a 54-year-old recent immigrant Arab laborer with ankle arthropathy and pain probably secondary to a symmetric peripheral neuropathy.

He focuses on the possible causes (hypotheses) for such a neuropathy, using the cues in his initial concept. The following list of hypotheses flashes through his mind, modulated by Mr. M.'s appearance and background:

1. infectious diseases of the Middle East such as bejel (a spirochetal disease related to syphilis) or leprosy
2. exposure to a toxin, such as petroleum distillates or solvents used in the lumber industry, or exposure to industrial chemicals used in the Middle East such as mercury or other heavy metals
3. a deficiency in nutrients such as B_{12} or folate (in a recent immigrant who has not yet learned to speak English and therefore may not be coping well with the change in cultures and available foods)

4. diabetes mellitus
5. spinal stenosis
6. side effect of over-the-counter medications or traditional homemade or herbal remedies

However, the clinician felt a vague sense of discomfort—as if he were making a basic blunder—but was unaware of its source. Further questioning and examination made each of these and several other hypotheses seem quite unlikely.

Finally, awkwardly, and without being sure why, the clinician asked Mrs. M.:

"Does Mr. M. ever drink alcohol?"

"He drinks all the time,' she responded in an exasperated tone. "I can't get him to stop even for a day."

"Really? Are you not Moslems, then?"

"No, we're Christians."

The clinician had been misled by a stereotypic bias of which he was not consciously aware: that Arabs don't drink alcohol. This assumption was perhaps arrived at by the following subliminal syllogism:

Moslems don't drink alcohol;
Arabs are Moslems;
therefore, Arabs don't drink alcohol.

Which led to

Mr. M. is an Arab;
therefore, Mr. M. doesn't drink alcohol.

The clinician was aware that some Arabs are Christians, but not aware enough to prevent this unrecognized bias from unconsciously obstructing his thinking and causing him to discard the hypothesis of alcohol-related neuropathy even before it reached consciousness.

This case illustrates well how bias can affect the initial concept. The clinician had repressed the obvious hypothesis of an alcoholic neuropathy that would occur to most clinicians seeing a 50+-year-old man with a symmetric peripheral neuropathy; a condition he had seen so often that he recognized it as familiar, without knowing why, in a patient he assumed to be a nondrinker. On reflection, after the patient encounter, the clinician became aware of some previously unconscious observations. For the first time he became consciously aware of the following perceptions:

- a ruddy complexion with erythematous cheeks, nose, and forehead
- smooth, shiny, very warm, somewhat livid skin with poor elasticity and a doughy feeling;
- a somewhat unpleasant odor of a sort that the clinician had learned to associate with chronic alcoholics

This unconsciously processed information, together with a characteristic pattern of sensory loss, arthropathy, and gait disturbance led the clinician intuitively to establish a fairly firm hypothesis, which then forced itself to consciousness.

Keeping the Initial Concept Flexible

The example of Mr. M. also illustrates the importance of keeping the initial concept plastic, of being able to review it, and to question observations, assumptions, and even hard data such as laboratory tests that don't fit the initial concept or are incongruent with other observations and facts. When you are working through a difficult case, you should take no bit of information as absolutely certain; each datum must be reviewed and reestablished.

In summary: Expectations based on previous contacts with patients usually determine which data are perceived and abstracted from all the information available at the beginning of the patient encounter. The clinician's interpretation of this data may be biased by unconscious attitudes and stereotypes. Watch this carefully.

DEVELOPING THE INITIAL CONCEPT

Tracking Patient Data

You may have had little to no patient experience at this point. When you encounter your patient, you may not have prior patient experience or extensive medical knowledge to bring to your aid in finding those pieces of information that could be important for your initial concept. At the start of your patient encounter you should pay systematic attention to all of the following methods of gaining data:

1. Carefully search for all the information you can gather from the patient's appearance, body language, age, sex, speech characteristics, and movement.
2. Determine any observations that might be useful about any of the people who have accompanied the patient: their attitude toward the patient, or toward you.

3. Try to determine if the patient is implying something other than what he or she is expressing verbally. Is there "more than meets the eye" in the patient's initial comments and actions?

4. Learn what you can about the patient's attitude toward you or toward the encounter itself.

5. If you already have found some ideas about what may be going on with the patient (see Chapter 4), look for whatever evidence that might substantiate those possibilities.

Practice looking, listening, (and smelling) in a thorough and consistent manner when you first confront the patient.

Initially you may find this a slow process, but it will speed up as it becomes habitual. By going through these steps you will avoid missing important pieces of information that may not be obvious but could be very helpful. As you develop more and more experience with patients you also will automatically seek particular vital items of information, as does the expert clinician. Discipline yourself now to be aware of all the available information and to think of how it could be helpful. Pull these potentially important items into your initial concept of the problem. Be aware of possible biases in your interpretation, and to the significance you attach to the data you have perceived. Are you making unwarranted assumptions? For example, a patient may appear depressed, and you may immediately think of him as "a depressed patient." Actually, the patient may not be depressed but may only *appear* depressed due to fatigue, or to an inability to smile. You might miss a chance to evaluate the patient accurately if you do not teach yourself to recognize the lack of a smile as a discrete

Try to avoid turning observations into diagnoses at this early stage.

piece of information, distinct from its emotional connotation. Patients with muscle weakness from myotonic dystrophy or myasthenia gravis that prevents them from producing a smile have been mistakenly referred to psychiatric care.

Facts vs. Diagnoses

In assembling information for your initial concepts, stick to observations *as facts* and try not to convert them into diagnoses: keep your patient data separate from your hypotheses. Also, be certain that you are not stereotyping the patient. Stereotypes can blind you to the real patient. Examine carefully your own attitudes, biases, and beliefs if you find that the patient or the patient's problem produces negative or hostile feelings you cannot readily explain: give the patient the benefit of the doubt.

TRANSLATION ERRORS

What does the patient really mean by the words he or she is using?

Since translation errors can occur at any time in the interview process, they are worth mentioning here. Do not assume you know what the patient means by the words he or she is using. Try not to substitute your own word, or a medical term, to describe what the patient is saying until you are sure you are right. The complaint of "numbness," for example—used by patients it could mean

- loss of sensation
- pins-and-needles sensation
- weakness without sensory change (believe it or not!)

Each implies quite different problems. Stick to the patient's words until you have clarified exactly what the patient means.

Another example is the complaint of "dizziness." Used by the patient the term could represent feelings of vertigo, syncope, or just light-headedness. Each has quite different implications. If the patient says "I'm dizzy," and you note "vertigo" you may be off to a bad start. Find out what the patient means.

A good way to avoid translation error is to ask yourself if you know exactly what the patient's complaint would feel like if you had it. Inquire until you know what it would be like to have the patient's symptoms.

In summary: Look at your patient carefully, listen carefully, and try to be as objective as you can about what you see and hear. Pull this initial information together, form your initial concept of the patient's problem, and your hypotheses will follow.

4

Generating Multiple Hypotheses

Hypothesis: "A proposition, or set of propositions, set forth as an explanation for the occurrence of some specified group of phenomena, either asserted merely as a provisional conjecture to guide investigations (working hypothesis) or accepted as highly probable in the light of established facts." (The Random House Dictionary, 2nd ed. New York, 1987.) These propositions spring into the clinician's mind almost at the start of the patient encounter. They guide the inquiry.

GENERATING HYPOTHESES

As soon as the clinician assembles the initial concept, a number of hypotheses jump into his mind. This occurs very early in the patient encounter. At least two hypotheses are generated—very often three or more, but rarely more than four or five. (Psychologists suggest that the short-term, or working, memory cannot hold more than five to seven separate ideas or concepts at once.) This may explain the upper limit to the number of hypotheses the clinician generates. There is evidence that the accuracy of these hypotheses and the promptness with which they appear in the clinical-reasoning process directly relate to the effectiveness of the clinician's evaluation of the patient. The experienced clinician does not often consciously search for hypotheses at this stage. As you will see, they come automatically through memory associations triggered by the initial concept. However, faced with an unfamiliar patient problem, the clinician may have to consciously search for hypotheses. This conscious search when the problem is difficult or obscure is part of the metacognitive processes that are discussed in Chapter 2.

The nature of the clinician's hypotheses is determined by the initial concept.

MR. HAWKINS

What were your initial hypotheses about Mr. Hawkins's problem? Write them down.

Relationship of Hypotheses to the Initial Concept

An illustration follows of how the particular hypothesis generated will depend upon the nature of the initial concept. If just one element were to change in your initial concept of a patient's problem, your hypotheses could change significantly. Work through these examples. Be sure to *write down* the hypotheses that come to mind when you read these initial concepts *before* you look at the lists. (If necessary, cover the lists with a piece of paper.) (Don't worry if you have just begun clinical work; do the exercises anyway—guess!)*

NINE EXAMPLES

1. A *young woman* complains of **sudden paralysis in both legs.** What comes to mind with this initial concept?

   Many clinicians would generate the following hypotheses:
   a. conversion hysteria
   b. multiple sclerosis
   c. acute polyneuropathy (Guillain-Barré syndrome)

   Now only *one* element in the initial concept described above will be changed.

2. A *middle-aged woman* complains of **sudden paralysis in both legs.** Now what comes to your mind?

   Faced with this, many clinicians would generate these hypotheses:
   a. vascular occlusion of the spinal cord
   b. spinal cord hemorrhage
   c. metastases to the spinal cord

   Now a *different* single element in the original initial concept described above has been changed.

3. A *young woman* complains of **slowly developing paralysis of both legs.** What are your ideas?

   In this instance many clinicians would generate the following:

---

* *Note:* It should be stressed that the power of this book will be diminished severely if the exercises in hypothesis development are just read, and not carried out as directed. (At the same time, students should be sure to keep a medical dictionary on hand to look up any unfamiliar terms as they encounter them.)

a. tumor compressing the spinal cord
b. motoneuron disease
c. progressive polyneuropathy
d. polymyositis

Let us try another example:

4. A *4-year-old girl* with **acute lower abdominal pain.** Again, what comes to mind with this initial concept?

Many clinicians may generate the following hypotheses with this encounter:

a. appendicitis
b. gastroenteritis
c. intussusception
d. abdominal migraine

Again, one element in the initial concept is changed:

5. A *22-year-old woman* with **acute lower abdominal pain.** Now what hypotheses come to mind?

Faced with this, a clinician might now automatically generate these hypotheses:

a. appendicitis
b. pelvic inflammatory disease
c. irritable bowel
d. urinary tract infection

Now two elements in the original initial concept are changed:

6. A *62-year-old man* with **acute *upper* abdominal pain.**

In this instance a clinician might generate these hypotheses:

a. peptic ulcer
b. cholecystitis
c. pancreatitis
d. atypical angina
e. mitral valve prolapse

How about another manipulation of an initial concept?

7. A *20-year-old male basketball player* has **episodic chest pain.**

   Hypotheses? They could be
   a. post-traumatic muscle injury or rib injury pain
   b. costochondritis
   c. pleurisy (viral infection)
   d. anxiety
   One change:

8. A *70-year-old male* has **episodic chest pain.**

   Now most of these hypotheses would be generated:
   a. angina
   b. esophagitis
   c. cholecystitis
   d. herpes zoster (and possibly an occult malignancy)

   Now, drop the **episodic** and substitute **acute.**

9. A *70-year-old male* with ***acute* chest pain.**

   Clinicians would generate most of the following, *totally different* hypotheses:
   a. myocardial infarction
   b. pulmonary embolus
   c. dissecting aortic aneurysm
   d. pneumonia

The initial hypotheses that pop into your mind, and into the minds of expert clinicians, are determined by the content of the initial concept. Your hypotheses will vary from those of others who read the same initial concept, because they are a product of your own experience and education.

Early Generation of Hypotheses

Hypotheses are generated early in the patient encounter. How early? The initial concept seems to cause hypotheses to be generated *almost at once* (Figure 3).

KEEPING EARLY HYPOTHESES BROAD

The clinician often keeps the initial hypotheses very broad and frames them in anatomic/pathophysiologic terms rather than as specific diagnoses.

FIGURE 3. With the formation of the initial concept, a number of hypotheses immediately spring to mind. These hypotheses guide the clinician's inquiry to get more information to shape the initial concept into a resemblance of one of the hypotheses (or to eliminate hypotheses).

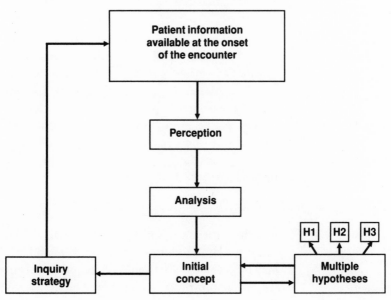

Each of the initial hypotheses might be elicited by any of a large number of disease entities. The clinician's initial questions will be designed to categorize the complaint (for example, chest pain) within one of these broad areas, and to rule out others.

MR. HAWKINS

The clinician's initial hypotheses for Mr. Hawkins were

1. visceral chest pain of cardiovascular or gastrointestinal origin
2. parietal chest pain such as pleuritic pain or musculoskeletal pain
3. psychogenic pain

Note here that the clinician generates another sort of hypothesis. The clinician's assumption (mentioned earlier) that the patient is sedentary, could be considered an hypothesis, but it is not one of the primary hypotheses used to guide the inquiry. Rather, it will provide the clinician with a useful way of organizing data relevant to certain diagnoses, to the prognosis, and later, to some treatment needs.

NARROWING DOWN THE HYPOTHESES

Broad initial concepts may contain too many hypotheses to be manageable, and may need focusing.

If the patient's complaint is too vague or if it suggests a large number of possibilities, hypotheses may be generated after some initial questions clarify the nature of the complaint. Questions will help focus the initial concept. For an example, assume that a patient says she has been more tired than usual in the last few months. Literally dozens of hypotheses are applicable to tiredness. You will need more information to determine what the patient means by "tired" and to narrow down the possible hypotheses. Questions such as "What seems to bring it on?" "What makes it better or worse?" "What other symptoms are associated with it?" "Does it come and go?" are needed to focus the initial concept better and to develop a more reasonable array of hypotheses to guide your inquiry. Since the possible hypotheses raised by such complaints as tiredness, dizziness, fatigue, abdominal distress, headache alone are legion, initial questioning is necessary to define the complaint more accurately so that the number of possible hypotheses becomes workable.

Initial questions that can clarify a complaint are described in detail in Chapter 6. These initial questions can be thought of as *dissecting questions* for a complaint. They will not only help you narrow down the possible hypotheses for the patient's complaint, they will also lead to a more accurate understanding of the patient's complaint and to the possible pathophysiological mechanisms responsible.

Hypotheses as Data Labels

Hypotheses serve as a collection of indexing keys for problem-solving. With hypotheses, the clinician transforms the ill-structured problem presented by the patient into a finite number of tentative, well-structured possible solutions to be investigated. Through the inquiry, the clinician attempts to examine the appropriateness of each of these hypotheses by obtaining more information from the patient.

Hypotheses are labels that refer to mental-information packages, and as labels they serve to guide inquiry. As a result they are hard to classify. They are unique file names for a collection of related clinical and basic-science data in the clinician's memory.

Some hypotheses are conventional *diagnoses,* and can be relatively specific.

- myocardial infarction
- Hodgkin's disease
- multiple sclerosis
- peptic ulcer

Some hypotheses may be *syndromes.*

- Horner's syndrome
- preeclampsia
- Ménière's syndrome

Some hypotheses may be labels for *pathophysiologic entities.*

- seizure disorder
- hypertension
- angina

Some hypotheses may propose or label *pathophysiologic* concepts.

- syndrome of inappropriate antidiuretic hormone release
- hyponatremia
- congestive heart failure
- demyelinating disease

Some hypotheses can represent *anatomic entities.*

- lateral medullary syndrome
- parenchymatous liver disorder
- lateral meniscus tear

Some hypotheses may label *etiologic* processes.

- viral infection
- syphilis
- nutritional deficiency
- drug toxicity

Some hypotheses may label *psychological* or *social* issues.

- conversion reaction
- family dysfunction
- marital discord
- litigation
- malingering

Hypotheses can also be any combination of the above. "Benign prostatic hyperplasia" can refer to an anatomic concept and a pathologic process. "Transverse myelitis" can be an anatomic concept, a syndrome, or a pathologic process, depending on how the term is intended by the person who uses it.

IDIOSYNCRACY OF HYPOTHESIS LABELS

It is better to look at hypotheses as *personal labels* clinicians have arbitrarily learned to use in order to identify and recall a particular collection of concepts and facts that they have learned about disease entities, pathophysiologic concepts, etiologies, and so on. Hypotheses are *idiosyncratic file names* for the individual who uses them. Although two different clinicians may call the same hypothesis by the same name, their definition or under-

Hypotheses are idiosyncratic labels for a personal collection of facts and concepts—a label for memory's filing and access.

standing of that hypothesis can be quite different. The facts that one remembers under a particular term is a product of education and past patient experience. Ask different clinicians what comes to mind with a particular diagnostic or anatomic term and you will observe great variation in the facts and concepts collected, depending upon each clinician's background. Hypotheses such as "emphysema," "peptic ulcer," or "transverse myelitis" can represent an anatomic lesion, a symptom complex, pathologic entity, or disease entity depending upon the clinician and the context of the patient problem. Gonorrhea can represent an infectious disease or an epidemiological/social problem. The name of the individual hypothesis means little in terms of its face value; you must know the facts and concepts that the clinician is connecting under the term used. Hypotheses can be best thought of as *individually authored titles* for a collection of data pulled together from the library of a clinician's long-term memory, data that are related to each other in various ways. These data are associated into various concepts, for which the hypothesis is a label. This collection of related data pulled together from long-term memory has been given such names as *prototype, pattern,* and *association set.* For our use, *hypotheses* serves well.

Hypotheses and Pathophysiologic Processes

Experts' hypotheses are basic-science stories from which they can recreate all the details of the patient's case.

The data contained in the hypotheses of expert physicians are often built around a basic-science story of physiologic or pathologic cause and effect that serves as a structure on which to hang all important facts about symptoms, findings, test results, age, and sex. This basic-science structure is easier to recall than a plethora of factual details, and can help bring those details to mind.

EXAMPLE

Multiple sclerosis offers a vast and complex set of clinical presentations, symptoms, signs, and disease courses. However, if the pathologic process and the locations of demyelination are kept in mind along with the physiologic effect of myelin loss, most of the symptoms, signs, and various courses of the disease can be reconstructed and remembered.

EXAMPLE

A clinician examining a short-of-breath woman entertained the hypothesis of pulmonary embolism. On stimulated recall (a technique used to analyze the reasoning process of clinicians while they are reviewing a videotape of a patient encounter they have just concluded) the clinician described a pathophysiologic model of oral contraceptives leading to deep venous thrombosis in the leg leading to emboli that were carried to the lung. This model guided the inquiry and problem-synthesis for the symptoms and signs that would support that hypothesis.

This basic-science-story background to hypotheses is something you must learn to develop, because it gives you the greatest flexibility in reasoning and allows you to reproduce a vast array of facts as needed. If you have a basic-science script for a specific disease process (the pathophysiologic mechanisms, anatomic changes, biochemical or immunologic events, etc., that occur in the disease) you can always reproduce the varied details of symptoms and signs appropriate to the particular patient problem. As you study about diseases in your patient work (see Chapter 13) be certain to work out this story in your own mind, and build on it as you run into other cases. In the course of a patient's illness, whenever symptoms, signs, or laboratory results do not fit this basic-science story, your script needs to be questioned and possibly revised (see Chapter 14). In some diseases the complete story is not actually known. In such a case, you should create a plausible basic-mechanism story that can explain most of the symptoms, signs, and laboratory tests, and use it until the medical literature comes up with a better script. Just realize that it is the "best fiction" until more facts are known, or until the patient's picture contradicts the story.

Broad vs. Specific Hypotheses

The collections of concepts and related facts pulled together under broad, less well defined hypotheses are themselves broad and less defined. For example, the hypothesis "something wrong with the spinal cord" is associated with the symptoms and signs of cord disease in general. A more specific hypothesis such as "subacute combined degeneration of the spinal cord" does not trigger an association with facts that deal with the spinal cord in general, but instead with specific concepts about symptoms and signs that would appear in this diagnostic entity, such as dietary and hereditary information. "Acute abdomen" is broad and inclusive and implies one set of concepts or facts about the symptoms and signs in the abdomen. In contrast, the more focused and specific "cholecystitis," "pancreatitis," and "Crohn's disease" imply a totally different collection of concepts and facts even though they are clustered around an acute abdomen. The clinician's hypotheses, generated at the outset of the patient encounter, describe possible causes for the initial concept as assembled. These hypotheses represent labels for collections of the clinician's knowledge at present.

Mr. Hawkins

With Mr. Hawkins, the clinician opens the history with the very broad question, "Can you describe to me exactly what your pain feels like?" (This very broad approach is based on Osler's dictum: Let the patient tell you the diagnosis.)

Mr. Hawkins responds, "I was digging up the garden after supper when I felt a pressure—like gas—right here." He holds his clenched fist over his lower sternum/upper epigastrium.

"I was able to belch a couple of times, but it didn't go away much. I broke out in a sweat and felt a little dizzy. I took some bicarbonate and tried to lie down, but felt like I had to be up and moving around. I feel like if I could belch some more that I would be okay."

What are your hypotheses now? Write them down.

STARTING THE INQUIRY AND REGENERATING HYPOTHESES

If you start your inquiry with broad questions (such as the one with Mr. Hawkins), the patient will usually give you information to answer many of the dissecting questions mentioned earlier in the chapter, saving you the time of asking them individually as well as giving you a relatively clear idea of his understanding of what is going on, his anxieties and concerns, and the questions that he wants you to answer and his expectations. It also enables the patient to give you raw data uncontaminated by any subtle leading cues and biases from your specific questions. You can then ask specific questions for areas not covered.

The Fixed Nature of Hypotheses During a Patient Encounter

Although hypotheses are frequently eliminated and replaced by new ones as the inquiry continues, each hypothesis itself is not changed or altered during its use in patient inquiry. The hypothesis is a fixed constellation of facts or ideas from the clinician's memory; when a hypothesis proves to be incorrect, unlikely, or too vague, it is replaced by another hypothesis. It is the clinician's internal representation or *synthesis* of the patient's problem under investigation that develops, grows, and changes during the clinical-reasoning process. The clinician attempts to put together an enlarging concept of the patient's problem from the data he has obtained following the initial concept, data obtained from inquiry guided by the hypothesis.

Hypotheses are unchanging guides and the patterns against which diagnostic decisions can be made. The clinician's problem synthesis, on the other hand, develops throughout the clinical-reasoning process.

Therefore, the facts in the patient's picture can be shaped to see if the findings on history and physical examination can match one of the entertained hypotheses closely enough to allow a decision on a diagnosis. You must develop your patient's problem with the data obtained from your inquiry to see if the problem can be made to resemble one of your hypotheses. However, care must be taken not to *force* the shape of the patient's problem to match one of your hypotheses. This will be dealt with in more detail in Chapter 7.

Hypotheses and Changes in Data

As you learn new facts about symptoms, signs, and disease processes from reading, lectures, and other experiences away from the patient, your collection of facts or concepts under a specific hypothesis label will change. As a result, the hypothesis will be a label for an improved set of facts or concepts the next time you recall it in your reasoning. For example, you may learn that a patient with a stroke due to vascular occlusion has headaches—a fact that you may not have learned from a previous patient experience, a lecture, a textbook, or wherever. If you talk to a neurologist or refer to the literature and find that headaches do occur in occlusive strokes, that fact will be added to your file collection. The next time you generate a hypothesis of cerebral vascular occlusive disease in your work with a patient, that fact will be included in the cluster of information you have underneath your hypothesis of "cerebral vascular disease." Conversely, cerebral vascular disease may be called up by association in an initial concept that involves the headache problem, where it may

New facts can change the facts or concepts collected under the hypothesis label.

not have been previously. With an appropriate experience a student may recall anthrax in a patient with malaise and dyspnea. Because of an unusual patient experience, a student may think of scleroderma in a patient with anorexia and fever. He might even think of a gastric-secreting tumor or multiple endocrine adenomata in a patient with symptoms resembling a peptic ulcer.

It is in this way that the student begins to develop the rich network of associations concerning facts, variations, and unusual hypotheses that characterize the expert. It's important, however, for you to realize when such associations are made that they may not represent the most frequent hypothesis for the presenting picture. It is the subtle and vast variations in medicine that are important in the expert's memory and that are learned in this matter. In fact, *all facts from basic science or clinical medicine that are learned around active problem-solving tend to be remembered well for a long time and recalled in active work with patient problems.* It is this important principle of educational psychology that can work well for you (and which motivated the writing of this book). As you learn, you must look into the frequency with which symptoms and signs occur in diagnostic entities, and the sensitivity and specificity of laboratory tests (Chapter 9).

The rich memory of the expert can be acquired only by active learning around patient problems.

Changing Hypotheses

Those hypotheses that *can* be rejected *are* rejected, and are often replaced by others. If none of the initial array of hypotheses can be either verified or rejected adequately by the inquiry, they are replaced by new ones. They are also replaced if unexpected information gained on history or physical suggests different possibilities. New hypotheses appear when new information indicates that some or all of the hypotheses entertained are no longer tenable. For example, a patient may present with recurrent dizziness as a complaint. The clinician's initial hypotheses might include Ménière's disease and brain tumor. However, subsequent information gleaned from the patient may indicate that he has diabetes and is taking insulin and that there is no evidence of any neurological symptoms or signs. Most of the hypotheses initially entertained would be dropped, and replaced by hypotheses such as hypoglycemia and cerebrovascular disease. Figure 4A demonstrates the replace-

Regeneration of hypotheses occurs when those considered cannot be verified, or when an unexpected piece of information suggests new possibilities.

FIGURE 4. (A) If in the inquiry process the initial hypotheses cannot be verified, or unsuspected data suggests new hypotheses, the first set is replaced by another set of hypotheses. (B) If one broad hypothesis is established, new hypotheses may be generated from it to carry the inquiry further to substantiate a more refined hypothesis.

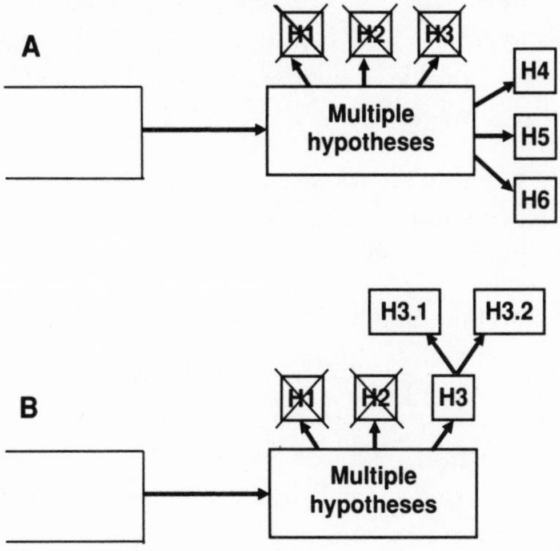

ment of hypotheses by a new set, when suggested by new information from the patient or by an inability to support hypotheses entertained.

The initial array of hypotheses is also changed if the clinician's more general or nonspecific hypotheses—as a result of information gained from inquiry—though established, are found to be too broad. At that time, the clinician generates a new set of more specific hypotheses to tune the investigation more finely (as seen in Figure 4B). For example, take an initial concept of a young woman with acute paraplegia. Broad hypotheses are usually generated initially.

1. conversion hysteria
2. something wrong with the nervous system

A broad hypothesis, once established, is replaced by more specific hypotheses to continue inquiry.

Guided by these hypotheses, the clinician may find on inquiry that the patient has abnormal plantar reflexes (Babinski's sign) and a distended bladder. The clinician now feels that the hypothesis of "something wrong with the nervous system" is confirmed, and immediately generates more specific hypotheses to investigate the nature of the patient's problem further. Such subsequent hypotheses might be

1. multiple sclerosis
2. acute polyneuropathy
3. hematomyelia

Let us take an initial complaint of hemoptysis, as another example. Initial broad hypotheses for hemoptysis could be

1. infection
2. epistaxis
3. tumor

Later, if fever, chills, and purulent sputum were found, more refined hypotheses would be generated, such as

1. infectious pneumonia
2. tuberculosis
3. bronchitis

Additional history indicates that the illness came on suddenly, about twelve hours ago, heralded by a rigor (shaking, chills). The patient looks toxic, is breathing at 27 times a minute, with decreased breath sounds, a pleural rub, and dullness to percussion in the left lower lung field. The list of hypotheses becomes further refined, and contains both very specific diagnostic possibilities that have a high probability because of patient characteristics and the clinician's recent local experience, as well as more general diagnostic groupings.

1. streptococcal pneumonia
2. Klebsiella pneumonia
3. Legionnaires' disease
4. mycoplasma pneumonia
5. viral pneumonia
6. other infectious pneumonias
7. noninfectious pneumonia

(The last two continue to be entertained to keep the clinician's mind open to unusual situations, and to enable him to respond to data that don't fit a common typical picture.)

The inquiry is now directed toward the most likely hypotheses, with questions to rule out the less likely.

As a further example, broad hypotheses generated initially with dyspnea or shortness of breath as a presenting complaint might be

1. cardiac problem
2. lung problem
3. anxiety
4. musculoskeletal disorder

When the clinician finds that the patient wheezes, more refined hypotheses such as

1. asthma
2. pulmonary edema
3. foreign body

would be generated in their place.

Grouped Hypotheses and the "Rare Bird"

The "rare bird" can ensure complete inquiry beyond the obvious.

Hypotheses generated during inquiry can be looked upon as a group. Except in the most obvious conditions, the clinician entertains at least two hypotheses to avoid coming to an obvious, but incorrect, conclusion about the patient. Clinicians are often chided for including "rare birds" in their group of hypotheses: rare, exotic conditions (such as the "oriental restaurant syndrome" for a patient with a headache). It has been thought of as the academic game of a medical faculty to enhance reputation or produce papers; however, the "rare bird" has a more useful function. Since "rare birds" are hard to establish on inquiry, their consideration forces the clinician to carry the investigation far enough to rule the "rare bird" in or out. This prevents the clinician from coming to an obvious, but possibly incorrect, solution. When you practice creating a group of hypotheses for a stomach or back pain, try to think of both common and rare causes to ensure a complete-enough investigation.

A good set of hypotheses causes the clinician

to consider all possible conditions that may be responsible for the patient's problem, particularly those that are prevalent, those that represent a serious threat to the patient's health or well-being, or those that are treatable. Again, experience helps the clinician recall appropriate sets of hypotheses for particular problems. However, one must be certain that hypotheses are logical and appropriate for the individual patient.

Hypotheses as a Net

A good set of hypotheses should form a net that will capture *all* the important data coming from the patient during inquiry or evaluation. Many studies have shown that if a finding bears no relationship to the hypotheses the clinician had in mind, the clinician will often *deny* that the patient gave that finding on history or examination. On review, it is usually discovered that the clinician was inquiring against a set of hypotheses in which the finding did not fit, and therefore did not perceive it. For example, a clinician evaluating a patient complaining of fatigue did not hear the patient mention that she had trouble carrying heavy books, because the clinician did not entertain a hypothesis of neuromuscular disease among the many he generated as a cause for her tiredness. If you are not looking for an item of information, you may not see it when it appears. This occurs again and again in formal studies of clinicians. They are shocked to see that they completely ignored an important fact. You simply cannot pay attention to all the data that comes from the patient during an encounter. Therefore, you must pay close attention to what the patient says or shows, write down in

If hypotheses do not form a good net, valuable data may be ignored. Attempt to cast a broad net for any symptoms or signs that do not seem to fit with your hypotheses.

your notes those items that do not seem relevant or that do not fit with your present hypotheses, and consider them on a later review. The best solution, however, is a complete hypothesis net. It is a good exercise to take some patient complaint and try to generate all the hypotheses possible about causes of that complaint.

BRAINSTORMING: HYPOTHESIS GENERATION AS A CREATIVE PROCESS

The generation of hypotheses is a creative, possibly right-brained, step in reasoning. It is an exercise in extending a range of hypotheses beyond those that might automatically be recalled. Experts constantly refer to their knowledge of pathophysiologic mechanisms to create novel or unusual hypotheses in difficult cases. You should engage in this creative brainstorming from the very beginning. Consciously reflect on which pathophysiologic mechanisms, altered anatomy, physiology, biochemistry, or behavioral dynamics might produce the initial concept. Use these possible mechanisms as a source of hypotheses. Also, think of patients or situations you have known before that might bear some relationship on the patient problem in front of you (this may not necessarily have to be a medical problem). Can you think of important possibilities that might be only vaguely suggested by the patient's information at hand? When you are presented with a difficult or unusual patient problem, broadly associate the patient's picture with everything you can possibly think of. Think of all the bizarre ideas, unusual conditions, or very "rare birds" that could be possible, no matter how unreasonable. These thoughts may bring out kernels for ideas, or trigger associations to a good hypothesis that you may have overlooked. *Exercise your creativity*. It will increase your ability to generate helpful hypotheses when your patient experiences or medical knowledge may be lacking. Do not restrict yourself to the few hypotheses you can hold in your working mind. Write them all down—ten, twenty, whatever! Try to assemble them into logical groups. When you are finished, review your list and pick up those few you feel are most plausible, those which pose the greatest threat to the patient, or those where treatability ought to be considered first in the inquiry. You can now appreciate why you often have to start with broad or general hypotheses. You can't remember more than a few hypotheses as you are working with the patient. Broad hypotheses are used to avoid having to remember many more specific hypotheses. Once a broad hypothesis— such as "something wrong with the nervous system"—is confirmed, many more specific areas can be considered. With complaints such as joint pain, weight loss or fatigue—which have numerous possible causes—you need to lump hypotheses into broader categories (collagen vascular disease, anemia, psychological problems, etc.), the more likely causes coming first in your inquiry.

When you are generating hypotheses in such a creative manner (especially to augment a lack of knowledge or clinical experience) try not to let your concern about medical knowledge restrict you. Be venturesome; you can always go to the books later to verify or develop your hunches.

Exercising creativity in hypothesis generation.

It can be very helpful in the early months of medical school to pretend that you have encountered your patient problem in an environment where no one is going to hold you responsible for specific, sophisticated, or complete knowledge of medical facts and terminology (that is, somewhere outside of your hospital, clinic, or medical school). This will help you "freewheel," expressing your thoughts in lay terms to see what you can bring to mind to explain the patient's presenting picture. I have seen students in high school, and even in the sixth grade, generate excellent hypotheses about patient's complaints on the basis of their own experience.

When the hypotheses you used with the patient problem seem inadequate to you, be sure to create an adequate list after you have learned what is wrong with the patient, and after you have studied the problem or talked with faculty. This educational approach, which is very powerful, will be considered in further detail in Chapter 14. Once you exercise your creativity in this manner, brainstorming will become a more automatic process and will serve you well.

Mr. Hawkins

What is your list of hypotheses for Mr. Hawkins?

The clinician's hypotheses at this point are

1. ischemic heart disease
2. acid peptic disease
3. esophageal spasm
4. other cardiovascular/respiratory pain

(i.e., pulmonary embolus, aortic aneurysm)
5. other gastrointestinal dysfunction (biliary colic, pancreatitis)
6. psychogenic pain

The clinician selects fairly specific hypotheses for what she considers to be the more urgent or probable problems, and continues to use broad categories to group other hypotheses. In this way she can continue to narrow the scope of each hypothetical category while keeping alert to information pertinent to all of the diagnoses. The clinician continues to use her hypotheses as a net, but rapidly closes that net in areas where she most likely expects to find useful information. By using general pathologic concepts, she is able to keep her hypotheses plastic and not focus prematurely on specific diagnoses. She mentally ranks the hypotheses in an order that directs the inquiry strategy.

The list is idiosyncratic to her personal style and experience. For example, another clinician might include alcohol-related illness as a separate hypothetical category, if it is a common factor in that clinician's patient population. This would guide that clinician to review the possible role of alcohol early in the inquiry.

The other general hypotheses previously considered, such as parietal chest pain, will remain at the back of the clinician's mind, to be triggered again into consciousness by any relevant bits of information.

5

Formulating an Inquiry Strategy

You have listened to your patient's initial complaints. They have been assembled into an initial concept. Hypotheses have popped into your head by association, or have been developed through a creative process. Another crucial step in the clinical-reasoning process now faces you—a step that often separates the novice from the expert. What information is needed to resolve the patient's problem to an appropriate hypothesis? What kinds of questions or examinations can most powerfully or efficiently separate the contending hypotheses? What do you do when the hypotheses do not seem to be verifiable? How can you be certain that other information—not related to your hypotheses, but important to the understanding of your patient's problem—has not been missed?

With almost any presenting patient problem, the clinician will need more information than is available at the outset to arrive at a diagnosis, or working hypothesis. He has to decide on the kinds of information from history, physical examination, and laboratory tests he will need to eliminate competing hypotheses and substantiate the correct hy-

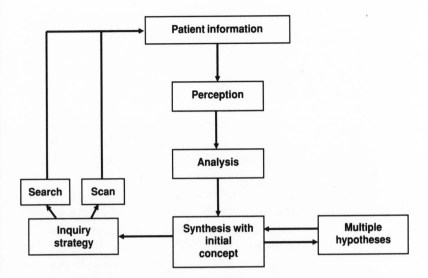

FIGURE 5. The clinician employs an inquiry strategy to obtain the information needed to verify or deny hypotheses entertained. If, in the light of the hypotheses, this new information seems significant, it is added or synthesized to the clinician's initial concept. The inquiry strategy employs both search and scan modes.

pothesis. Which of the initial tentative hypotheses is the most likely one to act upon? (As discussed in the preceding chapter, initial hypotheses are the propositions for the clinician to consider as possible or likely explanations for the patient's problem.) What does it take to rule out the incorrect hypotheses and establish the correct one? This diagnostic decision—choosing the correct hypothesis—is the vehicle for selecting the appropriate treatment for the patient. The sequence of questions that should be asked, and the items of physical examination that need to be performed to decide on the correct working hypothesis, is the *inquiry strategy* (Figure 5).

DESIGNING THE INQUIRY STRATEGY

Analysis and Synthesis

Inquiry produces data that are analyzed for their value relative to hypotheses, valuable data are synthesized into the initial concept.

Several kinds of thought processes seem to occur during the inquiry strategy. These might be collected under the labels *analysis* and *synthesis*. As the clinician inquires (asks questions and performs items of the physical examination), he analyzes the new data obtained about the patient for their value in supporting or denying the entertained hypotheses. Data found to be of value are synthesized into the *initial concept*. This synthesis of new data into the initial concept changes the initial concept into an ever-enlarging report on the patient's problem in the light of the clinician's hypotheses.

The inquiry strategy may be conceptualized as having four separate components, even though they are intermixed in practice: deduction, efficiency, search, and scan.

DEDUCTION

Deduction is the process by which you derive that data on history and physical examination that will help separate, support, or weaken your hypotheses. The success of deduction depends upon whether the information produced is a good test of one or more of your hypotheses. Does the new information support or deny the likelihood of one of your hypotheses? If the information provided by your inquiry does not do this and your hypotheses have remained essentially unchanged during the history and physical, the deductive logic of your inquiry strategy is poor. It is not uncommon to see students create an effective, nicely ranked set of initial hypotheses only to then ask a standard battery of questions they have learned to use on all patients—questions that are not necessarily related to their hypotheses in any way. If, after five to ten minutes of such *disengaged inquiry* they are asked what their hypotheses are, they will iterate their initial hypotheses ranked in their initial order of likelihood.

A most important function of deductive logic is to separate closely related or competing hypotheses so that the clinician can make a decision as to the more likely hypothesis. For example, a headache produced by certain brain tumors can be similar to a migraine in many respects. However, a brain-tumor headache will not change sides, whereas a migraine frequently does. A question about the headache changing sides would help separate these closely competing hypotheses. With chest pain, the clinician has to separate cardiac from noncardiac causes. "Does the pain vary with your breathing?"—Cardiac pain usually does not. The clinician may try to reproduce the pain by pressure or manipulation of the patient's chest: positive results would suggest noncardiac pain. If the clinician's inquiry discloses associated radiation into the left arm and symptoms of nausea, cardiac pain gains a high probability.

The rash and fever of measles and of Rocky Mountain spotted fever can be similar. A history of tick bite makes the latter more likely. A history of the rash starting on the head and spreading to the trunk and limbs, or the finding of Koplik's spots, makes measles the more likely candidate.

The young paraplegic woman described in Chapter 4 could be suffering from many conditions. A

Deductive inquiry counter-balances the creativity of hypotheses, deduction serves the critical, disciplined role in problem-solving.

question about vision producing a history of transient visual loss in one eye preceding the onset of leg paralysis raises the hypothesis of multiple sclerosis far above the rest. Clinicians who are trying to verify a possible hypothesis of multiple sclerosis invariably inquire intensively about early symptoms such as sudden loss of vision. This is deduction in inquiry. In your practice try to think of questions that will most effectively separate the hypotheses you are entertaining. What questions or examinations will help to establish one and weaken the other?

EFFICIENCY

Efficiency must be deliberately developed as an aspect of the inquiry strategy. It allows the clinician to economize on time, cost, and energy in her evaluation of the patient, and avoids unnecessary patient fatigue. It allows her to get the most valuable information in the time available. The strategies used in games provide a good analogy. The object of most games is to win in the shortest period of time; as a consequence, every play in a game should make progress towards winning—no unnecessary moves can be afforded. In clinical reasoning with patients, the cost of unnecessary actions in wasted time requires that all the clinician's actions should move toward identifying the patient's problem. In emergencies, the need to resolve the patient's problem quickly mandates that no unnecessary actions be taken. In the game of Twenty Questions, if you were told to name a large city in the United States, it would be doubtful that you would ask, "Is it Chicago?" or even, "Is it in Illinois?," as these actions are clearly inefficient—if pursued, such an inquiry could take all day. Most people would

If you cannot recall good strategies for inquiring about your patient's problem, then start to reason deductively against the hypotheses you are entertaining.

boil down the possibilities at the onset by a question such as, "Is it a city east or west of the Mississippi River?" or "Does the city have a population over one million?"

Studies of clinicians' problem-solving strategies demonstrate a similar behavior as they use questions that often relate to two or three of their hypotheses simultaneously, narrowing down the territory to be covered as quickly as possible. These studies have shown that the clinician with greater experience is consistently more efficient, and better able to arrive at a diagnostic conclusion with fewer questions, than the less experienced clinician.

In Chapter 4 we discussed the important balance between problem-solving skills and the richness of recallable factual knowledge and prior patient experiences. The expert can recall inquiry strategies that were successful with prior patients. The expert clinician, like the experienced game player, can get results in a few actions. He knows the territory. In your hometown, you know all the shortcuts to get wherever you want efficiently. You already are expert in finding your way in your "hometown" problems. The experienced clinician learns similar shortcuts for various problems. By contrast, if you are a stranger in town you do not know any shortcuts. However, it would be unlikely that you would wander about until the street you wanted appeared. You would inquire of maps or people, or make deductions about characteristic landmarks in your search. Both the strength of your reasoning powers and the range your experience and knowledge are important. Yet reasoning alone can get you quite far. When you are confronted by a patient, create an initial concept and generate some hypotheses: *think*. What is the best strategy to resolve the problem to its best hypothesis? Use the facts you have before you along with facts you can recall about similar problems, facts from basic science, pathophysiological facts—whatever you can muster—and apply them with good deductive reasoning skills. You can increase your efficiency by reviewing your inquiry strategy after you have diagnosed your case to judge how you could have been more effective in narrowing down your hypotheses.

MR. HAWKINS

What are the next two or three questions you will ask, or the next actions you will take, in evaluating Mr. Hawkins?

Write down your responses before you read on.

SEARCH AND SCAN

The deductive inquiry (designed to resolve entertained hypotheses) represents the search mode.

The inquiry strategy described up to this point is in the *search* mode. Information is sought to resolve the hypotheses that are entertained. Searching is a problem-oriented activity. Questions and examinations are carried out to get significant data. Clinicians will often obtain most of the information they need to resolve their hypotheses within the first one quarter to one half of the total time they spend in the patient encounter. A deliberate search for hypothesis-related information obviously occurs.

Another important inquiry method, employed for other reasons, is *scanning*. The radar beam methodically scans a segment of airspace to look for objects, not easily detected by other means, that could be of considerable significance. *Background, demographics,* and a review of *systems* (lists of complaints usually related to organ systems) all describe different areas in a scanning inquiry. The clinician scans by asking the patient questions about past illnesses and treatments, economic situation, family history, and social behaviors; by asking questions regarding dysfunctions in different organ systems; and by performing a routine or "screening" physical examination. Scanning, like radar, is performed to discover phenomena not easily detected by other means: in this case, facts, symptoms, or findings that either could relate to the patient's problem or represent another health problem that needs to be investigated as well.

Scanning is a non-hypothesis-oriented inquiry routine that complements the focused search of deductive inquiry.

Scanning is useful when the clinical-reasoning process has run aground. The scan may produce new information that can generate additional hypotheses or suggest new inquiry strategies to unstick the reasoning process.

Scanning may bail out the frustrated investigator who needs new ideas or approaches.

Scanning can build the clinician's confidence in the chosen hypothesis by uncovering supporting facts that were not directly sought. Sometimes scans can uncover unsuspected facts that weaken the suspected hypothesis. The scan can cause you to consider evidence that would suggest undiscovered alternatives. Scanning allows the clinician to buy time to ponder the patient's problem, review hypotheses, and review information. It is embarrassing to stop and stare at the patient while thinking or reviewing notes in the middle of the encounter. Studies have shown that clinicians frequently use scanning in this situation to ponder and yet appear actively involved in questioning the patient.

Scanning also buys time and builds confidence.

They appear just as intent and interested during this scanning as during their searching behavior. They frequently switch back and forth between scan and search, exhibiting no change in external behavior. It is valuable to memorize a repertory of questions about background, family history, and systems to recite when you want to pause over the patient problem, review the information you already have at hand, and possibly redesign your inquiry strategy.

Scanning allows the clinician to get to know more about the patient and his environment, and assures the patient that everything about him or her is being considered. Without doubt, getting to know the patient as a person facilitates rapport. Some clinicians scan *first* to get to know the patient and establish rapport, as a matter of personal style. They then move into a hypothesis-oriented search.

The degree of scanning used in any patient encounter seems to depend upon two factors. The first is the nature of the clinician. Some clinicians are quite content to problem-solve directly, confident that only a limited scan is needed to ensure nothing of importance is left out. Others feel strongly that a thorough database about each patient is important. Ultimately, the degree of scanning depends upon the available time. If the patient's problem seems to represent an urgent or emergency situation, little scanning occurs. Similarly, if there is little time available (as on a busy practice day or when the clinician is urgently needed somewhere else), scanning is attenuated.

In some instances scanning is a luxury to be used when time permits.

Memorize the standard review of systems early in your education. In addition to the useful functions described above, they provide a rich set of questions and examinations you can use in your search, guided by your hypotheses and your reasoning brain.

Thus far, the actions considered in designing an inquiry strategy have only included history and physical examination. Most laboratory tests and diagnostic studies, except those that can be performed during the encounter (such as electrocardiogram, blood count, catheterization), are performed some time after the patient encounter. There is a time delay, in both performance of the test and receipt of the test results. The clinician usually develops a strategy for using these tools when he decides upon the most likely hypothesis (or hypotheses) and management of the patient's problem. These actions—history, physical, tests, and diagnostic procedures—are usually aimed at further confirmation of the hypothesis chosen as the diagnosis, or to separate two or more likely hypotheses still felt to be likely. Some routine tests (such as blood count or urinalysis) also constitute scanning. Since information from tests is delayed, it does not affect the immediate diagnostic and therapeutic decisions you make about the patient. (These "long-loop" procedures are discussed in Chapter 9.)

Memorize the rituals of scanning so you can adapt them when you need them.

Hypothesis Generation vs. Inquiry Strategy

Hypothesis generation is a heady, creative process: brainstorming to come up with a good set of hypotheses. By contrast, inquiry strategy is a deductive, linear process requiring you to pick discriminating questions, examinations, or tests to rank your hypotheses. In other words, choosing actions that have the highest yield in discriminating among hypotheses. (This is possibly a left-brained activity.) The best guide to judging your progress in this skill is to examine how well your inquiry adds data needed to refine your hypotheses and enlarge your initial concept into a picture of the patient's problem that resembles one of your hypotheses well enough to be considered correct.

A good way to evaluate your progress is to note down the initial hypotheses that occurred to you when you first developed your initial concept upon confronting your patient problem. Then, after you have spent 5, 10, maybe 15 minutes asking questions, stop and ask yourself which hypotheses you are now entertaining. If you are still entertaining the same hypotheses, in the same order of likelihood as you had initially, then your use of deduction in your inquiry strategy is not very effective. As mentioned earlier, many students learn a set of routine questions that they ask every patient in almost every circumstance. This is a general waste of time, and does not stretch the brain.

> If your hypotheses have not changed as a consequence of your inquiry, your inquiry may be poorly designed.

Mr. Hawkins

The clinician interviews Mr. Hawkins while simultaneously examining him.

"Do you feel the pain anywhere else?"

"Yes. I have a heavy, achy feeling in my left arm, and in my lower jaw."

The clinician already has enough information to make ischemic heart disease the working diagnosis: it is the most probable problem, and effective treatment and the patient's well-being require the immediate institution of appropriate evaluation and management plans.

Other hypotheses are by no means ruled out, but they are moved toward the back of the clinician's mind because they are all less probable, and their management is generally less urgent. The clinician is already making management plans. These plans are not directed toward a specific diagnosis, but they are directed toward ensuring the safety of the patient, and toward rapid, definitive evaluation and treatment.

The clinician's list of hypotheses remains the same, except that ischemic heart disease is now divided into

recurring angina

unstable angina

coronary insufficiency

myocardial infarction, uncomplicated

myocardial infarction, complicated

The clinician asks some other quick, deductive questions to establish that other possibilities are less likely.

"Do you have any heartburn or burning in your chest?"

"No."

"Do you have any difficulty breathing?"

"Just a sort of heavy feeling in my chest, like it's difficult to get a good breath in."

This response adds some weight to myocardial ischemia and makes gastrointestinal (GI) pain slightly less likely. It also keeps the possibility of a pulmonary embolus in the clinician's mind.

"Have you felt any fluttering or pounding in your chest?"

"No."

The examination shows that there is no jugular venous distention above the sternal angle, that Mr. Hawkins's respiratory rate is 16 and unlabored, and that on auscultation he has no inspiratory rales, but a few scattered expiratory wheezes. His heart rate is regular at 85, with no extra systoles noted on examination or on the monitor. The first and second heart sounds are normal; there is no third heart sound, but there is a fourth heart sound. The clinician has also noted that Mr. Hawkins does not have an arcus senilis or ear-lobe creases (signs often associated with arteriosclerosis); these observations have no bearing on Mr. Hawkins's current management, but are helpful in developing the clinician's concept of Mr. Hawkins, and in forming an impression of risk and prognosis. The wheezes suggest the presence of some degree of smoking-related chronic obstructive lung disease. The clinician has also noted that Mr. Hawkins's QRS complex (a segment of the electrocardiogram) is not widened or of unusual form on the bedside monitor, and that there is only 2 to 3 mm of ST segment shift. ST segment shift on the monitor is nondiagnostic, but consistent with myocardial ischemia. The clinician feels that Mr. Hawkins's cardiac function is physiologically normal except for the fourth heart sound. She therefore tentatively concludes that Mr. Hawkins's myocardial ischemia is, so far, uncomplicated by rhythm or power problems.

At some point during the last few questions, the clinician has decided on initial management:

    admission to hospital

    electrocardiogram (ECG) and cardiac enzymes

    immediate drug treatment directed toward cardiac pain

    coronary-care protocol to deal with arrhythmias and congestive failure should they occur

    immediate cardiac consultation with a view to angiography and urgent definitive treatment as indicated by the angiogram: angioplasty, surgery, or biochemical clot lysis

Although these interventions will likely remain unaltered as additional information comes in, it is nonetheless very important to make the diagnosis as firm and as specific as possible, and to develop as clear and full a concept of the patient and all of the patient's medical problems as possible, to be able to provide optimal comprehensive care.

The clinician asks the emergency-room staff to do an ECG, draw blood, arrange a cardiac care unit bed, have arrhythmia treatments available at the bedside, start an IV, give the patient some sublingual nitroglycerin, and put in a call for the cardiologist. While these actions are being accomplished, she begins to ask Mr. Hawkins scanning questions, simultaneously continuing the examination.

REDESIGNING THE INQUIRY STRATEGY

Frequently, as mentioned in Chapter 4, new hypotheses have to be generated because the inquiry was unsuccessful or because one hypothesis in the first set is found to be correct but too broad to direct further inquiry. Before treatment can be entertained, a new rank or more finely tuned, specific subhypotheses is needed to select a more specific diagnostic entity. For the same reasons, you may need to redesign your inquiry strategy during your encounter with a patient in response to a change in a hypothesis or to a realization that your inquiry is going nowhere. When inquiry has led you into a blind alley, when the hypotheses cannot be resolved to any satisfaction, or when no worthwhile information seems to be available, it might be valuable to switch to a *scanning* mode of inquiry. Figure 5 summarizes the search and scan options used by the clinician.

MR. HAWKINS

Scanning questions produce the following useful information:

Demographics and habits: Mr. Hawkins is indeed sedentary, takes no regular exercise, has smoked 1½ packs a day for 35 years, and has 2 to 3 drinks with dinner most evenings.

Family history: He has a stable marriage and two grown children; both parents had myocardial infarctions before the age of 65, though both are still alive and otherwise healthy; two of his three siblings have high blood pressure, and one of these is obese, has adult-onset diabetes, and has had a heart attack.

Systems: He has frequent dyspepsia and sometimes heartburn. The epigastric pain of the dyspepsia is quite different from his current pain. He coughs up 1 to 2 table-spoons of thick white sputum each morning. For the past year he has had some difficulty in initiating urination and some dribbling following.

Medical history: He was treated for "ulcer" ten years ago, when his dyspeptic pain was much worse. He has been on 50 mg daily of hydrochlorothiazide for high blood pressure for the past 15 years, but he only takes it intermittently. He was also on Inderal, but quit taking it because of the lack of energy it caused. His blood pressure generally runs in the 140–150/90–100 range.

The clinician notes mentally that she has already ordered blood tests appropriate to this information (i.e., serum potassium, blood sugar, lipids, hemoglobin, urinalysis, and oxymetry).

The clinician does not have a firm diagnosis. She does have a well-ordered, structured list of hypotheses and an initial management plan that both ensures the patient's well-being and will probably establish a specific diagnosis, as well as define the altered anatomy, physiology, biochemistry, and severity and prognosis of that diagnosis.

6

Applying Appropriate Clinical Skills

History and physical examination are the clinician's investigative tools in the scientific approach to the patient's problem. The scientist reads, then experiments. The detective questions, then uses laboratory results. The clinician takes a history, and then examines. For each type of professional, the first phase of investigation is usually free or flexible, the latter more ritualistic and modified to the needs of the problem at hand.

Clinical skills are the psychomotor skills for data-gathering to carry out your inquiry strategy in the scientific approach to your patient. These skills of history-taking and physical examination, (see Figure 6) are usually well covered in medical schools. There are excellent books and videotapes that can help you learn these techniques. Only those aspects of clinical skills that relate to your clinical reasoning will be considered here.

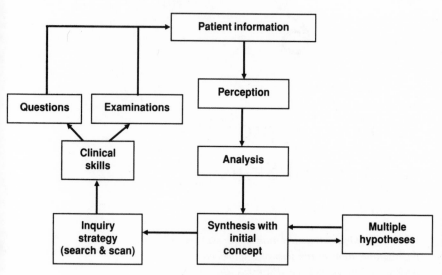

FIGURE 6. Clinical skills are investigative tools directed by the inquiry strategy.

THE HISTORY

Your history-taking has to adapt to the particular communication problems presented by your patient. The interview of a parent of a confused or an elderly patient, of someone with poor skills in your language each requires an adaptation of the usual interview techniques.

Open questions are needed to determine the real nature of the patient's problem.

As mentioned in Chapter 4, the use of open-ended questions such as, "Tell me why you came to see me," or, as in the case of Mr. Hawkins, "Can you describe to me exactly what your pain feels like?," used early in the interview of the patient, will encourage the patient to expand on his complaints. Such questions imply no particular information from the patient, leaving the patient free to relate any concerns, feelings or symptoms. As a consequence, open-ended questions provide a treasure chest of information from which to draw cues for the initial concept of the patient's problem. Again, subsequent *direct* questions dissect out the specific characteristics of the patient's individual complaints, and allow the clinician to gain the type of information needed for hypotheses. These are search questions, questions that dissect out the nature of the patient's complaints or symptoms. These direct questions usually cover the following areas:

Reason for the encounter: Why is the patient here at this particular time? Remember, few patients present to you until they have treated themselves, talked to friends or relatives about their problem, or sought other health practitioners. It is important to determine exactly what has occurred to finally lead the patient to you.

Direct questions dissect and elaborate on the patient's complaint

Onset of the problem: When did the patient first notice any unusual symptoms? It is important to establish the true onset. The patient may only be aware of his symptoms now that they are full blown. ("Did you ever have anything like your present difficulty earlier?") If the patient's problem is episodic, when did he have the earliest episode? The time of the onset can put a completely different perspective on the problem. If a patient complaining of recent incoordination tells you that he has been clumsy for many years, what may have seemed acute is now possibly chronic or even familial. Little pains in the chest may have preceded an anginal attack by a long time.

Events surrounding the onset: What was the patient doing when the problem or symptoms began? Where was the patient? This can be very helpful in establishing causation for the problem. That the onset of the symptoms followed exercise, eating, or an emotionally or physically trying time can support an appropriate hypothesis array.

The quality and intensity of symptoms: What do the symptoms really feel like, and how severe are they? Encourage the patient to use his own words freely, to use any adjectives or similes that come to mind. Words are often inadequate to describe symptoms, and the clinician must be sensitive to this quandary. Suggest a range of possibilities—as, with a headache; "Aching?" "Jabbing?" "Burning?" "Deep?" "Pressure?" The clinician must always try his best to understand the nature of the symptoms the patient is feeling. Can you imagine yourself having the patient's symptoms? Translation error (discussed in Chapter 2) is often committed by clinicians at this point. The clinician should not try to reduce the patient's complaint to a convenient medical term, as the term might not be accurate. Can you really understand the quality of the symptoms? Verify what the patient means by the particular words used in describing symptoms.

The severity of symptoms is impossible to measure objectively. Nevertheless, it is important to estimate severity when at all possible. Nonverbal cues of distress observed as the patient describes complaints can help in this estimate. However, everyone varies in their sensitivity and responsiveness to pain or discomfort. The best way to estimate severity is to determine how the symptom changed that patient's behavior or daily activities. Was nausea severe enough to stop food intake? Did abdominal pain stop activities? Did headache cause the patient to leave work and go to bed? Another technique is to use numbers. If a patient is weak, for example, ask him to consider normal strength as 10 and then to give you a figure between 0 to 10 to estimate his present strength. This is useful with pain, strength, and many other symptoms.

Associated symptoms: What other symptoms occurred with the patient's principle complaint? This includes a review of those symptoms most apt to occur with that complaint, considering the initial hypotheses that you generated.

Temporal profile: How the severity of the patient's illness changed over time is often the best clue to the disease process responsible for the patient's symptoms and signs. What is the course of the illness? Did it evolve slowly or rapidly? Did it plateau, or does it fluctuate? Does the symptomatology come in discrete episodes? All disease processes have characteristic modes of onset and characteristic temporal profiles (Figure 7 graphically demonstrates these profiles, and Figure 8 characterizes different profiles for some common infectious diseases.)

Sequence of symptoms. During the illness or in a discrete episode of the illness, were there warning symptoms? As the episode or illness

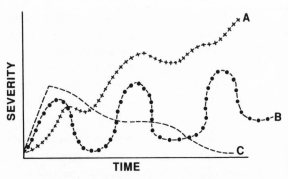

FIGURE 7. Characteristic temporal profiles for neurological diseases. (A) A relentlessly progressive course can suggest neoplastic or degenerative disease. (B) Recurrent attacks with increasing deficit between attacks can suggest demyelinating or vascular disease. (C) Sudden onset with progressive clearing or worsening can suggest infections and vascular disease. (Adapted from *Guide to Neurological Assessment* by H. S. Barrows. J. B. Lippincott Company, Philadelphia, 1980.)

evolved, which symptoms came first? . . . second? What is the relationship of symptoms to each other? This information can give clues to the underlying pathophysiological mechanisms.

Pneumococcal pneumonia usually starts with a chill and severe rigor, followed by fever and cough; later, rust-colored sputum is produced. Viral pneumonia, by contrast, may begin with upper respiratory or gastrointestinal symptoms, and the patient may suddenly deteriorate days later with a bacterial superinfection.

Localization of symptoms: Where are the symptoms located in the body? Do they radiate? Do the symptoms occur in synchronization with any other symptoms in other locations?

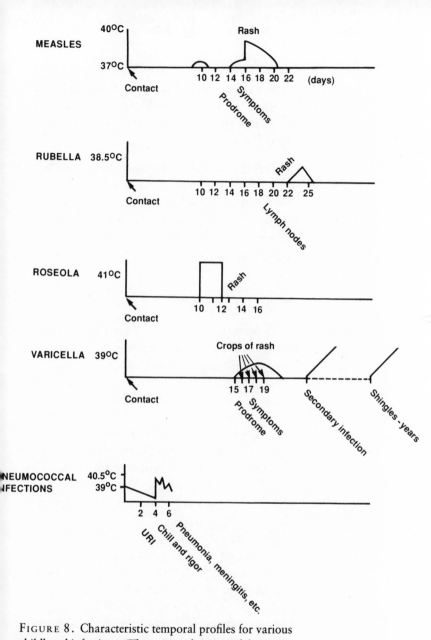

FIGURE 8. Characteristic temporal profiles for various childhood infections. (The pace and timing of the symptoms and signs of an illness can help the clinician separate various hypotheses.)

93

Physical or emotional stress, illness, or injury preceding the problem: This information can provide clues to the possible mechanisms responsible for, or factors that may aggravate, the patient's problem.

Relieving factors, aggravating factors: Is the patient aware of anything that modifies or worsens any symptoms, such as particular daily activities, foods, environments, lights, noises, or seasonal changes? This can provide further clues about the pathologic mechanisms responsible.

Open vs. Closed Questions

Closed questions may influence the patient's answer, and elicit incorrect data.

In dissecting out the true nature of the patient's symptoms with direct questions, you must be sure to avoid suggesting answers. Do not ask, "Are your headaches throbbing?" The suggestible patient, or the patient who is not able to describe his symptoms verbally, may well agree with you. At least offer the patient options such as "Are your headaches constant? Throbbing? Or do they feel some other way?" Avoid suggesting an answer. The more open question—"What are your headaches like?"—would produce an even more accurate and richer response.

Another common error is to limit an initially open question by suggesting alternatives. "Have you ever had trouble with your vision (*open*) such as, spots before your eyes or loss of vision (*patient is limited to only two choices*)?" The broadly inquiring first part of the question about vision might bring any kind of visual complaint to the patient's mind. If, for example, the patient had episodes of double vision in the past, he would more than likely mention this. However, the alternatives tagged on to the end made it clear that the clinician only wanted to hear about spots or visual loss. It is often helpful to see yourself interviewing a patient on a videotape to discover these common errors. In fact, a videotape gives you a valuable and objective look at yourself, and how you come across to patients. It can be very helpful in developing your clinical skills.

Working with Baffling Cases

The list in the preceding section only partially covers the question that will help you gain the information you need to resolve your hypotheses and assemble an accurate synthesis of the patient's picture. Such dissecting questions need to be augmented by appropriate questions about health, family, (including family illnesses) work, friends, and particular questions concerning the patient's own perceptions and opinions about his complaints.

The types of questions listed above, in addition to producing valuable information about the patient, will help you inquire about a patient's problem *even when you are at a loss to understand what is going on.* These questions will give you a working database about even totally unfamiliar patient problems, and can guide you when you have difficulty in coming up with adequate hypotheses, a significant number of hypotheses, or a worthwhile inquiry scan. As you ask these questions, information may come out that will prime your reasoning process.

Intelligently used dissecting questions can help work through an unfamiliar or baffling problem.

As mentioned in the preceding chapter, you should memorize routine questions about the symptoms produced by various organ system dysfunctions and social problems so that when you are in a blind alley or wish to round out the picture of the patient you can scan for new information. Routine systems questions will help you buy time to ponder over the patient's problem.

Reviewing the history with the patient.

A valuable technique used by many clinicians is a review of their understanding of the patient's history with the patient near the end of the interview. Doing this allows you to make certain all the information you have noted is correct and that you understand correctly what the patient has described. This review often stimulates other memory associations or new insights on the part of the patient. It also reassures the patient you have understood his or her problem.

Mr. Hawkins

The clinician asks the following specific questions of Mr. Hawkins to provide very specific bits of information to round out her concept of the patient.

"Do you have any allergies to medications or to anything else?"

"I am allergic to erythromycin."

"What happened when you took erythromycin?"

"After about the second tablet I got pain in my stomach and nausea and started throwing up."

Patients are likely to classify almost any drug-related adverse medication event as an "allergy." It is important to find out specifically what happened. Particularly in the case of very important drugs such as betalactam antibiotics, failure to differentiate between life-threatening reactions and nuisance side effects can prevent the patient from benefiting from an important medication.

"Do you take any other over-the-counter drugs or medications?"

"Oh, I take a couple of aspirins a day. Actually, they are coated aspirin so they don't bother my stomach so much. I've heard aspirin prevents heart attacks and a doctor once told me it may keep me from getting gout again. Oh, I forgot to tell you I had gout in my left foot three years ago."

Patients often forget to tell you things. Reiterating similar questions and engaging in cross-examination may help to complete the picture.

"Do you sleep well?"

"Yes."

"Do you have much life stress to deal with?"

"Not really. My job is a little aggravating sometimes, but not bad. My wife and I get along pretty well. I'm generally pretty happy with life."

The clinician then verbally reviewed her patient concept as developed to this point with Mr. Hawkins.

"Now, as I understand it, you were working in your garden after supper when you developed a heavy, severe, fairly constant pain in the middle of your lower chest associated with sweating, nausea, belching, and a feeling of lightheadedness. The pain radiated to your left arm and your lower jaw and you felt quite restless with it. You have had ulcer-related pains in the past but never anything that felt like this. You don't have any other unusual or abnormal feelings or sensations now. In the past you have had an ulcer, and one episode of gout. You have hypertension treated in the past with hydrochlorothiazide and for a while with Inderal. You have smoked a pack and a half a day for 35 years. You drink about three drinks a day, and you take coated aspirin every day. You don't take any regular exercise, you don't follow any particular diet, and you are not particularly stressed. Both of your parents had heart trouble before they were 65, as has one of your brothers. Is that all accurate?"*

"Yes, I think so."

"Have you ever had your cholesterol checked or been checked for diabetes?"

"No, I don't think so."

"Is there anything else that might be important that I should know?"

Concurrently, the clinician was completing her physical examination. She was looking specifically for physical findings associated with coronary artery disease, diabetes, peripheral vascular disease, alcoholism, chronic ob-

---

* This represents the clinician's *problem synthesis*. It contains significant data related to the hypotheses entertained and is organized in a sensible cause-and-effect relationship. Problem synthesis is described in Chapter 7 (and a more elegant synthesis of Mr. Hawkins presented).

structive lung disease, acid peptic disease, gout, and hyperlipidemia. Otherwise it was a cursory screening examination. The clinician carried out some procedures (such as checking a couple of reflexes) simply because patients often expect them to be part of a "complete exam." Other pertinent examinations were purposely deferred. For example, the clinician did not do a rectal to examine the patient's prostate, or check for occult blood, because the reflex vascular response to this examination is undesirable in a patient with ischemic chest pain.

> "Did the nitroglycerin we just gave you have any effect on your chest pain?"
> "Oh, maybe it relieved it a little bit, but not very much."

The clinician considers this to be an item of significant *negative* data. The clinician has also noted that the cardiogram just completed has an abnormality consistent with her working diagnosis: 4 mm of ST segment elevation in leads V1–V4—significant *positive* data.

The Physical Examination

It is said that 90% of a diagnosis is based on the history alone. Most studies continue to bear out the truth of this statement. In fact, the physical examination is often used only to confirm what has already been decided during the history. After the patient interview, an experienced clinician can usually tell you exactly what he plans to do and

The physical examination is a ritual, modified to substantiate conclusions on history and to scan for undetected findings.

what he expects to find on his physical examination of the patient. He usually has only a few particular examinations in mind, examinations that are needed to confirm his diagnostic decision. The rest of the physical examination is usually a scanning procedure, a quick routine aimed at finding unsuspected problems.

The physical examination is an opportunity for "hands on" contact with the patient, and to many patients is an expected part of any appointment with a clinician. Realizing this, many clinicians perform a physical examination when they do not expect to find anything. It is important that you know how to perform a routine scanning physical examination. By definition, this is the examination that should be performed on a patient who has no complaints or physical findings.

Again, you should learn how to *search* by means of physical-examination techniques when an abnormality is found. You need to be able to confirm the abnormality you discovered by alternative examination techniques, if possible. If a finding is present, what else can you learn about the abnormality? What additional observations are possible? What will enhance the finding? What other findings may be associated with it? Search techniques are needed to focus on the finding, whether it is elicited pain, a skin lesion, an abnormal movement, a lump on palpation, abnormal sounds on auscultation, something seen in the otoscope or ophthalmoscope—whatever.

Learn the best way for you to carry out your examinations, and always do them that way.

Your physical-examination techniques should be consistent. Decide on the way you are going to test strength, tone, sensation, palpate, auscultate, perform reflexes, and so on. Always perform these techniques in the same manner. In achieving consistency you will develop an awareness of the range of normal responses and be able to pick up subtle abnormalities early. Apparent abnormalities can be produced both by examiner error and change in examination technique. *With poor technique you can produce findings where they do not exist in the patient.*

Clinical skills are your data-gathering tools in your scientific approach to the patient. Use them to carry out your inquiry strategy. However, if you do not know what you are looking for or what you are seeking, you run the risk of not seeing or hearing abnormalities that might well be in front of you. Experience with students and studies of physicians have repeatedly demonstrated that symptoms or signs may appear in the patient encounter and pass totally unnoticed by even the most careful clinician *if he or she is not looking for them.* Clinical skills must be employed as the handmaiden of your hypothesis-guided inquiry. This is the reason for rich hypotheses, and for a carefully designed inquiry strategy. This is also why it is a good policy for you to decide what it is you expect to find on physical examination once your history has been completed.

Although it is traditional and convenient to take a history first and then do a physical examination, there is no set reason why this should be true. In fact, there are good reasons why it should not be true. You should go after the data you need in the best sequence to narrow your hypotheses efficiently and effectively. Oftentimes the patient may present a symptom that can be interpreted in several ways, and a brief examination can suggest the right interpretation. Could morning headaches be due to high blood pressure? Find out by taking

If you don't look for something you won't find it. You must always have a good idea of what you are looking for on physical examination.

the blood pressure. What does the patient mean "by a lump in my throat?" Is there a lump, or is there difficulty swallowing? Feel and find out. The patient feels as though his heart were beating rapidly or jumping in a funny manner, but is not sure. Feel the pulse, or listen to the chest and find out. The patient says his arm is clumsy, yet he cannot describe clearly whether it is weakness or incoordination. Do an examination and find out. An item of the physical examination at the right time can save you from a long interview down an unproductive channel. This interdigitation of history and physical works both ways; it is often efficient to scan or ask further questions while examining the patient.

7

Developing the Problem
Synthesis

As the inquiry continues and more data are obtained from the patient, the clinician adds the data he believes to be significant to the information assembled in the initial concept. To do this, the clinician has to notice the new data and analyze them for their value in resolving hypotheses. This continual synthesis of new data is the problem synthesis. *Analysis and synthesis are at the heart of all logical inquiry.*

REVIEWING THE PROCESS

Guided by his multiple hypotheses, the clinician designs an inquiry strategy to ferret out data needed to analyze and resolve the patient's problem. By means of his clinical skills, he gathers data to carry out the inquiry strategy and to add to the initial concept. Eventually this hypothesis-driven data-gathering process should allow the clinician to decide upon the more appropriate final hypothesis to facilitate the correct management of the patient. This is the summary of the patient encounter.

A quick summary of where we have been so far.

103

During this cyclical process, new hypotheses may be generated and new inquiry strategies designed to arrive eventually at diagnostic and therapeutic decisions.

Adding New Data

Are new findings on history and physical accurate?

As this process cycles through the interview and examination of the patient, new information is produced beyond that originally assembled into the initial concept. These new data need to be analyzed in several ways before being added to the initial concept. Are they accurate? Are they to be trusted as a true indication of the patient's situation? Can they be trusted as a sign of an abnormality? Confidence gained in your clinical data-gathering skills through practice and increasing patient experience will help you in making this decision.

Evaluating the New Data

Are new findings significant in terms of the hypotheses entertained?

Are the new data significant? Do they support or weaken any of the guiding hypotheses? This decision depends upon knowledge about, and experience with, the hypotheses entertained. If you are not sure of this in your work with the patient, *write* the facts or data down for later analysis on a convenient note pad. Significant or hypothesis-related data can be considered positive or negative. Positive data are symptoms or signs that you would expect to find if a particular hypothesis were true, and which therefore support the hypothesis. Negative data are expected facts that are not present, facts that would be expected if the hypothesis were true and which therefore weaken the hypothesis

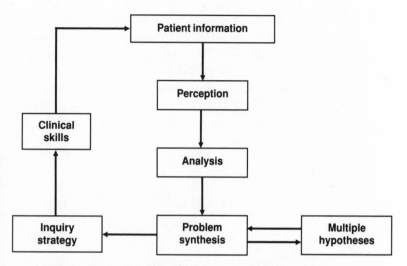

FIGURE 9. As the inquiry, guided by the hypotheses, progresses, the newly perceived data that are analyzed as significant against the hypotheses are continually synthesized to what was the initial concept, and is now the growing problem synthesis which plays a central role in the whole process.

by their absence. You suspect migraine headache, yet the patient does not have the nausea that usually accompanies migraine associated with his headaches. That is a significant negative item. Since most clinicians ask questions or perform examinations aimed at several hypotheses at once, one piece of information may have different consequences for different hypotheses—positive for one and negative for another. However, once analysis suggests that the new fact is significant, positive or negative, *it must be added to the initial concept.* This addition of significant new data to the initial concept enlarges and shapes the picture of the patient's problem. As an ongoing process in clinical reason-

The problem synthesis is an enlargement of the initial concept.

ing, this continual and cumulative assembly of significant data into a growing picture of the patient
as the inquiry proceeds is the *problem synthesis*.
Figure 9 shows the central role of the problem
synthesis and its reciprocal relationship to hypotheses. The initial concept, developed early in the encounter, was actually the earliest form of the problem synthesis.

SYNTHESIZING THE PATIENT PROBLEM

The Role of Deduction

The basic plan of your patient inquiry is to see
how closely new data can shape the problem synthesis to resemble one of the hypotheses entertained
in your mind. In Chapter 4, hypotheses were described as individually authored file names that
label a rich collection of related information in
the clinician's mind—information, acquired from
learning and experience, that is unique for the individual. Within that fixed mental collection of facts
and concepts are the usual symptoms, signs, laboratory results, and pathophysiologic or clinical
concepts that the individual clinician feels belong
to the hypothesis (whether the hypothesis is a diagnosis, a syndrome, an anatomic or physiologic de-
rangement, whatever).

Since the inquiry strategy is aimed at supporting
or denying hypotheses, by application of clinical
skills the clinician will attempt to discover how
much of those recalled facts or informational bits
subtended under the title of each hypothesis can

be discovered in the patient. The significant data that are added to the initial concept represent part of a growing collection of information about the patient, acquired for the most part from recalled hypothesis-related information in the clinician's memory. This addition of significant data forms an enlarging problem synthesis, which can be best thought of as an attempt to see if the shape of the patient's problem does in fact match the shape of one of the entertained hypotheses closely enough for it to be accepted as a diagnosis.

EXAMPLE

As an exercise to demonstrate how hypothesis-guided inquiry produces new significant data that needs to be synthesized into the problem synthesis, let us take the case of the young woman with an acute paraplegia from Chapter 4. Imagine that the clinician entertained these hypotheses:

The hypothesis-guided inquiry process shapes the patient's problem in the direction of an entertained hypothesis.

1. multiple sclerosis
2. spinal cord lesions
3. conversion hysteria

Let us assume the clinician would recall these facts under the hypothesis *multiple sclerosis*:

- This disease occurs in younger people with greater frequency in women.
- The illness comes in separate attacks.
- There are usually symptoms and signs indicating lesions in more than one place in the nervous system.
- The symptoms and signs are usually associated with lesions in the white matter of the nervous system, such as in the spinal cord, optic nerve, brain stem, or cerebellum.

- Acute visual loss ("optic neuritis") may be a characteristic of the first attack.

Also, let us assume that the clinician would recall this fact under the hypothesis *spinal cord disease*:

- There are usually "long tract signs" such as increased tendon reflexes, bladder dysfunction, extensor plantar responses (Babinski), sensory loss below the segmental level of the lesion.

Under the hypothesis of *conversion hysteria*, the clinician recalls the following:

- It occurs more commonly in young women than in young men.
- Patients show little distress (*la belle indifférence*).
- Sensory or motor losses are nonanatomic.
- There is usually secondary gain achieved by the disability; the symptoms accomplish something for the patient as an unconscious mechanism.

At the beginning of the interview, the clinician notices that the patient is very anxious about her paralysis. This fact is added to his initial concept because it represents a significant *negative finding* for conversion hysteria, where little distress is characteristically shown. The problem synthesis in the clinician's mind at this point would be

An *anxious* young woman with an acute paraplegia.

The clinician has enlarged the initial concept by the term *anxious,* which begins to shape the patient problem further. He may then try to challenge

The clinician uses a hypothesis-guided search inquiry to find significant data that will shape the problem synthesis to resemble one of the hypotheses entertained.

this hypothesis of conversion hysteria even further, and on interview try to establish the existence of an uncomfortable or difficult life situation in which the paralysis provided secondary gain for the patient. As this is occurring in the emergency room where the implicit contract denotes urgency, the clinician would probably not stay at this task very long. With this patient, such a brief line of investigation would reveal no positive information. In fact, the patient could become irritated with such psychiatric implications to the questioning. The clinician would then add more in the way of significant facts to his problem synthesis:

> An anxious appearing young woman who, *without prior evidence of emotional stress,* develops an acute paraplegia.

To test spinal cord lesion, the clinician asks about bladder dysfunction and finds that the patient had a urinary urgency yesterday and has not urinated today; because the clinician integrates history and physical for efficiency, he palpates his patient's lower abdominal area and finds a mass consistent with a distended bladder. (Notice how the inquiry strategy produced data that affected two hypotheses at once. Bladder dysfunction is very likely in spinal cord disease and highly unlikely in conversion hysteria. The clinician would then place conversion hysteria as a less likely hypothesis and place spinal cord disease as a more likely hypothesis.) In this process the problem synthesis grows further with new additions of significant data.

> An anxious appearing young woman, who without prior evidence of emotional stress, but with *urinary*

urgency yesterday, develops an acute paraplegia. *On examination she has a distended bladder.*

The clinician then examined the patient for reflex and sensory changes to determine if there were "long tract signs" that could further support the hypothesis of a spinal cord lesion. This examination did show these signs, giving further support to the hypothesis of spinal cord lesion. Multiple sclerosis was not weakened as a possibility since it could involve the spinal cord. However, as a result of this new significant information, the problem synthesis is further shaped in the mind of the clinician.

An anxious appearing young woman, who without prior evidence of emotional stress, but with prior urinary urgency, develops an acute paraplegia. On examination she shows a distended bladder, *extensor plantar responses, hyperactive tendon reflexes in the legs, and a loss of pin sensation below the umbilicus.*

Notice how this creative shaping by inquiry and synthesis has produced a picture of the patient that can be compared with and tested against the facts and concepts gathered underneath an entertained hypothesis. Much unrelated data brought out during the inquiry, felt to be insignificant, were not added. Unresolved is the question of multiple sclerosis, as the patient picture fits both the hypothesis of spinal cord lesion and the hypothesis of multiple sclerosis. The clinician therefore asks the patient about prior episodes, such as loss of vision, that might suggest multiple sclerosis as the correct

The shape of the problem synthesis is critical in making a choice between competing hypotheses.

hypothesis. He finds that, indeed, the patient did have transient visual loss in the past that had been treated with "little white pills." This visual loss has cleared for the most part at the present time. Now the problem synthesis in the clinician's mind would be the following:

> An anxious appearing young woman, who without prior evidence of emotional stress, but with prior urinary urgency, develops an acute paraplegia. On examination she shows a distended bladder, extensor plantar responses, hyperactive tendon reflexes in the legs and a loss of pin sensation below the umbilicus. *One month ago she had a transient loss of vision which is slowly clearing.*

The match between the clinician's personal concept of multiple sclerosis and the way he has synthesized the patient's picture is close enough in his mind to accept multiple sclerosis as the final working hypothesis, or diagnosis. The clinician now moves on to hospitalization and treatment, choosing those tests and procedures that might further establish the hypothesis and determine appropriate treatments.

This clinician had decided to take only a brief look into emotional problems. If he had chosen to spend more time, despite the emergency-room setting, he would have learned about a missed menstrual period for six weeks and a great concern about a clearly unwanted pregnancy in this single woman. If this data had been added to the patient's early problem synthesis, the clinician would have felt that conversion hysteria was the more likely, if not the actual, problem. Subsequent neurological findings may have led to spinal cord lesion or multi-

The picture synthesized by the clinician depends on the investigation carried out, even though the hypotheses may be the same.

ple sclerosis, if the clinician had paid close attention to the examination findings.

The Problem Synthesis as a Representation of the Patient

The preceding case and many others have been presented[*] to a variety of clinicians over the years in the form of standardized or simulated patients. The reasoning, as described, has been seen time and time again with a variety of clinicians. Patients are seen in the light of the problem synthesis. The problem synthesis is *not* an objective picture of the patient, it is a deliberately created synthesis, encompassing only those attributes that seem relevant to the entertained hypotheses. This underlines the critical role of hypotheses: poor hypotheses can lead to incorrect conclusions.

Poor hypotheses can also lead to an incorrect problem synthesis.

EXAMPLE

The initial concept of a "62-year-old man with acute upper abdominal pain (from another patient in Chapter 4) leads to this initial set of hypotheses:

1. peptic ulcer
2. cholecystitis
3. pancreatitis
4. atypical angina

The clinician's memory collections associated with the first three hypotheses would cause him to note that the patient lies very still with his legs drawn up, suggesting peritoneal irritation that the clinician notes as being possible also in the first three hypotheses. This finding also tells him that

[*] By Howard Barrows.

the patient's problem is both serious and urgent. The problem synthesis develops from the initial concept in the following way:

> A 62-year-old man with acute upper abdominal pain, lying very still with legs drawn up.

Notice that the clinician did not state this finding in the problem synthesis as "with signs of peritonitis," as this type of thinking does *not* belong in the problem synthesis; it is a diagnostic impression. Peritonitis could have been one of the entertained hypotheses, and if established might then be replaced by the first three hypotheses mentioned above. The clinician asks about the quality of the patient's pain and learns that it is sharp, constant, severe, and knifelike. Although anginal pain usually radiates to the left arm and neck, the clinician asks about pain radiation and finds that it goes around the patient's right side into the back. This question has a strong effect on the competing hypotheses, as it eliminates angina as a concern, decreases the likelihood of peptic ulcer or pancreatitis, and strongly suggests of cholecystitis. It also raises a concern for renal colic, a hypothesis that replaces angina. The problem synthesis might be as follows:

> Diagnostic labels do not belong in the problem synthesis. The problem synthesis should only contain a meaningful narrative of symptoms and signs.

> A 62-year-old man with acute, sharp, constant upper abdominal pain that radiates to the right back, who is lying very still with legs drawn up.

The *regenerated* hypotheses would look like this:

1. cholecystitis
2. renal colic
3. peptic ulcer
4. pancreatitis

5. peritonitis (secondary to 1, 3, or 4, or of another cause)

Examination for signs of peritonitis—guarding, rebound tenderness, and referred tenderness—produces negative results. Peritonitis is ruled out and pancreatitis is judged unlikely. To pursue the possibility of cholecystitis the clinician palpates the upper right quadrant of the abdomen and finds tenderness, which is a positive significant finding for the diagnosis of cholecystitis. Now the problem synthesis has enlarged further.

> A 62-year-old man with acute, constant right upper quadrant pain and tenderness radiating to the right back, without guarding, rebound, or referred tenderness but with right upper quadrant tenderness.

Note that the clinician has dropped the finding of "lying still with legs drawn up" since it was of no further use after he eliminated peritonitis in his thinking. Further examination produced many confirmatory signs for cholecystitis. There was none of the costovertebral angle tenderness that is found in renal colic. The clinician could next return to the history and *search* for more information to increase his confidence in the decision for cholecystitis. At the end of the encounter, after many questions and examinations, the problem synthesis has grown to

> An obese, 62-year-old Navajo man, with acute, constant right upper quadrant pain and tenderness radiating to his right back and shoulder. Onset occurred with a heavy meal of fried food, followed promptly by nausea and repeated vomiting. He is not jaundiced, has a low grade fever and a positive "Murphy's sign" [splinting of respiration with right upper quadrant pain].

Note that obesity and absence of jaundice were obvious at the outset but were only noticed later as relevant findings, and then added to shape the problem synthesis to match the selected hypothesis. Also note how the clinician employed an efficient inquiry strategy at the outset to rule out the most potentially dangerous conditions. All the niceties to support cholecystitis came later.

If you read this clinician's written consultation or case write-up you would assume he got all those items in the initial history. *The case write-up is no place to learn about clinical reasoning.* Even at this point the clinician has not decided on only one hypothesis. Alternatives are still possible, but they are more refined.

The case write-up (or clinician's pathologic conference) does not illustrate clinical reasoning.

1. cholecystitis
2. carcinoma of the gall bladder
3. hepatitis

The Problem Synthesis and Clinical Reasoning

The problem synthesis is central to the scientific analysis and synthesis of the patient's problem, and is an essential segment in good clinical reasoning. Whenever an experienced clinician is asked about a patient, no matter how complex the patient problem, or how long he has worked with it, he will invariably provide a capsule summary containing all the significant data he is working with, similar to the statements in the preceding section. This summary rarely contains unnecessary data and rarely leaves out any significant data. The data is usually organized in a way that suggests the underlying pathophysiology of the disease process

The problem synthesis is the key to effective communication between clinicians.

as the prior examples show. Hearing this synthesis, another clinician can easily comment on the first clinician's diagnostic ideas and suggest his or her own, as well as other inquiries that might be relevant to those hypotheses. *This is the all-important problem synthesis.* It is a key factor in communication between clinicians.

By contrast, when asked to describe a patient encounter, students will frequently begin to recite a rambling narrative of all the facts they obtained on history and physical examination. No attempt is made to sort out and organize the wheat from the chaff, the significant hypothesis-related facts from the total information base. When students present a patient case in this manner to clinical faculty, the faculty clinician usually will feel impelled to go to the patient, take another history and undertake another physical examination to "better understand" the problem. The faculty clinician was not able to appreciate the *shape* of the patient problem because it was not synthesized in the student's description. The faculty clinician had to create his or her own synthesis to think about the patient.

The development of the problem synthesis is the key to developing secure clinical-reasoning skills.

During many years of work with medical students, it has become abundantly clear that once students can develop a problem synthesis, their clinical-reasoning skills take a significant jump forward in effectiveness. In addition, the students' ability to communicate quickly and easily with faculty about their patients improves immeasureably.

CLARITY

It is difficult to be confident in (or tolerant of) orally presented cases by students or postgraduate clinicians unless the presentation has the characteristics described above. In a large clinic or patient service, a long, rambling narrative takes up time, and to most clinicians is aggravating and boring because it does not get to the heart of the matter. Hearing a student or postgraduate clinician present a clear-cut problem synthesis along with a final working or diagnostic hypotheses allows another clinician to quickly understand the problem and determine what additional items of information may be needed to check out his or her own particular hypotheses generated by the offered problem synthesis, to see if they agree with that of the student or postgraduate clinician.

In working with clinicians who spontaneously verbalize their thoughts as they work along with the patient, you can hear their problem synthesis growing in their thinking along with their hypotheses.

The problem synthesis plays an important reciprocal relationship with hypotheses in the clinician's working memory. As we have seen, the facts put into the problem synthesis are, for the most part, a result of hypothesis-oriented inquiry. The clinician attempts to see if the problem synthesis, as it gains informational shape, resembles any of his generated hypotheses. In some instances, as the patient's problem takes shape in the problem synthesis, it may become clear that none of the hypotheses are satisfactory, and new hypotheses need to be generated. Also, during inquiry, data may be elicited that seem unrelated to the present group of entertained hypotheses, and yet appear significant. Because of its apparent significance, the clinician adds the information to the problem synthesis. This may change the shape of the problem synthe-

The relationship between problem synthesis and hypotheses.

The problem synthesis provides the key element in distinguishing between pattern recognition and the scientific clinical-reasoning process.

sis, and require new hypotheses. The hypotheses and the problem synthesis are counterpoised in the clinical-reasoning process.

The clinical-reasoning process has been described by some as *pattern recognition*. Pattern recognition implies that the clinician's multiple hypotheses are patterns, and he tries to see if the patient's problem can match one of them through his inquiry. This implies that the clinician inquires of the patient without creating a separate patient pattern (called here a problem synthesis). The only conclusion the clinician can make at the end of such an inquiry—without a central problem synthesis of the patient—is that the patient does or does not fit one of the hypotheses entertained. No central theme is developed to test hypotheses or to change to new, more adequate hypotheses. As a result, the pure pattern recognizer tends to force the patient to fit the disease. Without a problem synthesis, the hypotheses entertained in the clinician's head are his only reference.

The problem synthesis itself may have to serve as the evaluative or diagnostic statement for the patient's problem. This is more honest than accepting a hypothesis that truly does not fit.

It is possible that the patient being investigated may represent a unique or unusual problem, and it may turn out that the clinician can generate no satisfactory hypotheses. In this instance, the problem synthesis, having encapsulated the shape of the problem, can serve as the working diagnostic statement at the end of the inquiry. The clinician can use this statement as a focus for subsequent study or research to find better hypotheses. This is the way new diseases and syndromes are found. Many who think they use pattern recognition actually employ the clinical-reasoning process, but are unaware of the existence of the problem synthesis. Remember, so much of the clinician's thinking oc-

curs in a twinkling that it can be largely unconscious.

ADHERENCE TO BASIC-SCIENCE FACTS

As mentioned in Chapter 4, the expert organizes
his patient problem synthesis around a basic-science scenario or pathophysiologic story. A clinician
examining a short-of-breath woman and entertaining a hypothesis of pulmonary emboli would see
if the synthesis could be built around a scenario
of oral contraceptives leading to venous thrombosis in the leg veins, with emboli to the lungs causing
shortness of breath. You should try to organize
your synthesis around basic mechanisms of anatomy, physiology, biochemistry, and pathology in
a pathophysiologic sequence. If no hypotheses can
be verified, you are left with a pathophysiologic
story for your patient that can suggest possible
treatment options on the basis of the assumed
pathophysiology.

The synthesis is best developed around a basic-science story.

As in the initial concept, the problem synthesis
contains data from many sources: letters of referral, records, notes, test results, comments from
the patient (either spontaneous or in answer to
questions), the patient's demeanor, and so on. It
would be an impossible task for you to remember
all of the information that flows from the patient;
instead you select only the significant data for your
problem synthesis. (However, be sure that you do
not overlook any significant useful data—positive
or negative—that may relate to your hypotheses).

Having recognized the central role of problem
synthesis, how do you apply this knowledge to
your clinical-reasoning skills? In your own encounters, once you have pulled together the important

information from the patient and his setting into an initial concept, generated multiple hypotheses, designed an inquiry strategy, employed your clinical skills to fulfill the strategy, and begun to analyze new data for their significance in support of your hypotheses, you still must add that significant data to the initial concept to start the problem synthesis. *Stop frequently in your ongoing work with the patient and consciously review your problem synthesis.* Deliberately look at it, develop it, and compare it with your hypotheses.

In your patient work, be certain you are always carrying a clear mental image of the patient's problem.

SIGNIFICANCE

In your recurrent ongoing mental review of your problem synthesis, make sure that the data are significant. Keep your problem synthesis concise by avoiding the thoughtless addition of insignificant data. However, at the same time be careful not to leave any important data out. If you feel that you might be doing this, review the data you have in your memory about your hypotheses. Also, be sure you have not influenced your possible future diagnostic decisions by entering a piece of data into the problem synthesis that is an interpretation of data and not the data itself. Remember the problem synthesis for the 62-year-old man with acute upper abdominal pain. The clinician did not add the diagnostic statement "peritonitis or peritoneal irritation" to the problem synthesis. Instead, he noted that the patient lay on his side with his legs curled up. This prevented the clinician from being biased about possible alternative hypotheses for the pain. Does your problem synthesis say that the patient is depressed, or *appears* depressed (a big difference)? Does your problem synthesis say that the patient has "pleurisy" or

The criteria for an effective problem synthesis.

pleuritic pain; "stroke," or *right hemiplegia;* "migraine" or *recurrent headaches;* "anginal pain" or *chest pain?* Keep diagnostic labels, diseases, syndromes, and eponyms out of the problem synthesis. The problem synthesis should contain significant data, not interpretations or mini-diagnoses.

MR. HAWKINS

The clinician made a telephone call to consult with a cardiologist about Mr. Hawkins. "I'm seeing a patient whom I believe to have new onset myocardial ischemia." This opening statement presents the consultant with the working hypothesis or diagnosis, and cues him to evaluate the clinician's problem synthesis as a basis for that diagnosis. In presenting the problem synthesis, however, the clinician gives only uninterpreted raw data. The initial statement orients the consultant to confirm the clinician's initial impression of myocardial ischemia, and to help the clinician work through the more specific differential diagnosis of specific ischemic syndromes. The time and energy saved by obviating a broader differential will be useful in their discussion of further investigation and management.

The clinician presents her problem synthesis:

Mr. Hawkins is a 54-year-old, white, married postal worker, with no prior cardiac history. He experienced the sudden onset of severe, heavy, constant, substernal chest pain associated with nausea, lightheadedness, sweating, restlessness, and radiation to his left arm and lower jaw while working in the garden after supper, two hours ago. The pain continues unabated and was unrelieved by nitroglycerin. He has a positive family history, hypertension, gout, and is a smoker. On examination his blood pressure is 140/80 at 85 per minute. He has no evidence of congestive failure or dysrhythmia. He has a fourth heart sound and stigmata of hypertension, COPD [chronic obstructive pulmonary disease], and peripheral vascular disease with copper wiring and AV [arteriovenous] nicking in his fundi, scattered expiratory wheezes, and absent dorsalis pedis and posterior tibial pulses. His cardiogram demonstrates 4 millimeters of ST segment elevation in V1–V4.

ASSEMBLING DATA TO ARRIVE AT THE FINAL STORY

In your recurrent ongoing mental review, you should also see if you can assemble the data you have synthesized into a meaningful pathophysiologic story. Does that story encompass all the data? What unexplained data are left? What data are still needed to establish the story? Is the evolving story consistent with the hypothesis or hypotheses entertained?

Including Background Data

Keep your eyes open (ears and nose as well) for significant data that may not be hypothesis-related. Use your note pad to aid your memory.

There will always be data you will want to include as background data about your patient. Also, there will be some patient data that might have significance, but that you may not be willing to put into your problem synthesis as it is not really hypothesis related, but that could suggest new hypotheses should you end up in a blind alley. There will be data, presently unrelated to your ongoing data search, that appear during the patient encounter that you know you will want to explore later in the interview or examination, to dissect more deeply. There will be considerable data you will need to learn about the patient as a person—such as values, beliefs, and life situation—not only for their potential diagnostic value, but because of their value in making appropriate management decisions. All these instances underline the important role of your note pad. For example, be sure to jot down any treatment ideas or questions that you will want to pursue eventually but which would interfere with the flow of your inquiry strategy were you to pursue them directly.

IDENTIFYING THE FINAL PROBLEM SYNTHESIS WITH THE PATIENT

The problem synthesis *is* your representation of the patient. When you are finished with your encounter, the final shape of the problem synthesis is your concept of the patient problem. If your problem synthesis matches one of your hypotheses closely enough for you to select that hypothesis as a diagnosis, remember that the hypothesis is still only a convenient label. *The problem synthesis is your patient.* The detail of your problem synthe-

The problem synthesis, not the diagnosis, is your patient.

sis must be recorded, and kept in mind at all times. As new data become available they may change the problem synthesis in a way that would suggest a change in your diagnosis.

Keep practicing the careful development of your problem synthesis. Keep looking at the relationship of the problem synthesis to the hypotheses. Use the problem synthesis as a key to changing hypotheses, just as you use the hypotheses as a key to inquiry. Eventually synthesis will become automatic, and you will notice a marked improvement in your reasoning.

8

Continuing the Clinical-Reasoning Process

The important segments of the reasoning process have been described as isolated but related segments. Clinical reasoning is a dynamic, cyclic, reiterative process in which observation, analysis, synthesis, deduction, induction, hypothesis generation, hypothesis testing, inquiry-strategy design, and the skills of examination are all interrelated.

CLINICAL REASONING AS A DYNAMIC PROCESS

The evaluation of the patient by the use of clinical reasoning—the scientific method of the clinician—is a dynamic process. It is easy to lose sight of this in the previous chapters, as we have dealt individually with the important segments of a process: (initial-concept formation, hypothesis generation, inquiry-strategy design, clinical-skills application, and problem-synthesis development). However, the clinical-reasoning process is a continuous, cyclic activity. Figure 10 depicts these elements as a cycle. The hypotheses serve as guides,

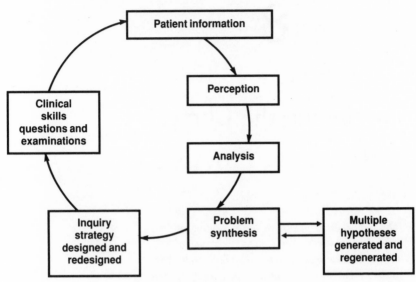

FIGURE 10. The clinical-reasoning process as a continuing cyclical process.

the inquiry strategy directs the inquiry process, selecting the correct clinical skills to serve as information probes or data-gathering tools. The problem synthesis serves as a continually updated progress report or work record of the significant facts gathered in the encounter with the patient. The data that are gathered are analyzed for relevance and then added to the problem synthesis as appropriate. Blind alleys in the inquiry process or unexpected changes in the problem synthesis may cause the hypotheses to change. Also, hypotheses may change to direct the inquiry towards more defined diagnostic entities. The hypotheses may change when the clinician is unable to resolve existing hypotheses; these new hypotheses may alter the design of the inquiry strategy. The inquiry strategy may move from search to scan to find new information or to buy thinking time. Around and around this process goes until the clinician is satisfied that he has resolved the patient's problem as far as possible in the time available.

If the above summary statement seems correct and understandable to you, please go on. If it does not seem correct or understandable, please review those chapters that relate to the segment summaries you don't agree with, or you don't understand.

Forming the Initial Concept at the Start of the Patient Encounter—Review Chapter 3.

Generating Multiple Hypotheses—Review Chapter 4.

Formulating an Inquiry Strategy—Review Chapter 5.

Applying Appropriate Clinical Skills—Review Chapter 6.

Developing the Problem Synthesis—Review Chapter 7.

THE INDIVIDUALITY OF
PATIENT PROBLEMS

Every patient is unique, and a source of infinite data. The clinician is trying to obtain those data that best help him understand, and therefore, manage his patient's problem. As symptoms, feelings, life experiences, nonverbal information, and information from the physical examination unfold before the clinician, various amounts of puzzling, confusing, and unexpected data may emerge. Initially the patient may seem to present a straightforward problem, easy to evaluate: a splinter in the finger, a sore throat, a headache, a minor back pain. But as the clinician delves into the problem, it may turn out to be quite different, with surprising turns, complications, combined problems involving multiple organ systems, psychiatric or psychological problems, financial and social complications. The combined flexibility, rigor, and quality of multiple hypotheses combined with problem-oriented inquiry and analytic/synthetic reasoning allows the clinician to adopt a logical approach to the complexities of the patient's problem.

STRATEGIES FOR DIFFICULT PROBLEMS: CHANGING YOUR THINKING

Ten Steps to Take

What will you do when you hit a blind alley in this process? What will you do when you can't seem to resolve a problem, when no hypothesis seems correct, or when you can't decide between several hypotheses? A number of strategies may be adopted when this (not uncommon) situation develops. Some of these you can do during the encounter, others when you can ponder the patient's problem afterwards.

1. *Review and recalculate your hypotheses.* Maybe a new one will come to mind. Perhaps your hypotheses are too specific or too vague—juggle them!

2. *Review the problem synthesis and see if some reorganization of the data will change it and suggest new hypotheses or approaches.* There are a couple of ways to do this.
   a. Can you state the problem synthesis in other words?
   b. Can you eliminate some of the data in the problem synthesis? Perhaps some information is unnecessary, and only clouds the real shape of the problem.
3. *Analyze the problem synthesis and see if it suggests two problems that might be separated, each requiring a separate set of hypotheses and inquiries.* Patients can have both measles and a broken leg. The presence of data from one condition may obscure the presence of another. One example of this is a young woman who developed a progressive symmetrical weakness of all four extremities due to polymyositis. Because an attack of childhood encephalitis had left her without any significant residual symptoms except for bilateral extensor plantar responses (Babinski's sign) not previously recognized, she presented a paradoxical collection of physical findings that made it difficult for examining clinicians to realize that her progressive symmetrical weakness in the extremities was due to muscle involvement, and not to some process in the central nervous system. It is common for elderly patients to present with multiple new problems that may or may not be related to each other. An elderly man with known congestive heart failure, palpitations of the heart, nausea,

dark urine, diarrhea, and muscle weakness represents such a challenge. Investigation of this man revealed problems of renal failure, hyperkalemia, and digitalis toxicity. The renal failure was an independent problem made apparent clinically, as were the other new problems, by the regimen used to treat his congestive failure. A 32-year-old woman with tiredness, poor sleep, diarrhea, heat intolerance, nervousness, and a late menstrual period was another challenge: is this one problem or more? It was found that her husband had left her and that she had physical signs of depression and hyperthyroidism. Did the hyperthyroidism precipitate the marital stress, or vice versa? Which problem is responsible for the amenorrhea?

4. *Analyze your inquiry strategy.* Perhaps it needs to be changed. If you review the hypotheses, they might suggest another approach to data collection, or suggest information that might better separate your hypotheses.

5. *Scan.* Look for new cues to rejuvenate the hypotheses and the problem synthesis.

6. *Review data already available from other sources: referral letters, prior medical records, laboratory data, and so on.* Originally you may not have reviewed the material carefully enough to notice potentially significant data. However, after you have worked with the patient for a while, this significant data may be more obvious to you because of hypotheses you are now entertaining.

7. *Find out what your patient thinks is going*

on. Ask your patient if there is other information that you should know. It is amazing what ideas a patient can produce that you may not have thought of. The patient has lived with the problem and, chances are, has thought about it a lot.

8. *Organize the data in the problem synthesis some other way.* Review it backwards from the present to the past, or start from childhood and come forward. Start from the onset of a different symptom than the one you had chosen originally. A new juxtaposition of facts could reveal unrecognized relationships. Draw diagrams of the data you have in the synthesis and note their relationship to each other.

9. *Present the problem to someone else: a colleague, another clinician, a nurse, a student, a spouse, or a friend.* Frequently the act of consciously verbalizing your thoughts gives you new insights. The very act of formulating the synthesis aloud encourages you to rethink it, and new connections or insights may occur. In addition, the person you're talking with may stimulate your thinking by his or her insights, concepts, or questions. This is a powerful method. Don't fail to use it whenever you're really puzzled.

10. *Take a break.* Pull together what you know in written form, under the hypotheses you have at present. Decide on appropriate tests that might help you. Treat the most obvious diagnostic possibility or the one that may represent the most undesirable possibility in terms of outcome or complications. If this is not possible, then treat the symptoms

you can without unnecessary risks or complications, and arrange to see the patient later. How much later depends upon your concept of urgency. In this way, you are able to do some study and, more importantly, to let the problem simmer on the back burner of your mind for a while (as discussed in Chapter 2). Time is a powerful weapon, and many problems will resolve to a more readily recognizable stage upon its application.

EXAMPLE

A 4-year-old Mexican American girl presented with new onset of fever for six hours, headache, sore throat, and abdominal pain. Initial cues indicated a girl who was well nourished and well cared for, but acutely ill. Initial general hypotheses consisted primarily of febrile infectious illnesses including

- upper respiratory illnesses such as otitis media and viral or bacterial pharyngitis or tonsillitis
- lower respiratory illnesses such as bronchitis and viral or bacterial pneumonia
- gastroenteritis
- appendicitis
- urinary tract infection
- meningitis

Lower-probability hypotheses at the back of the clinician's mind included bacteremia or sepsis secondary to focal infection and chemically or environmentally induced pyrexia.

The girl and her mother reported no prodromal symptoms, no prior significant medical history, and no other current symptoms. The family had wintered in Mexico, and had returned to the United States three months before. No one had been ill in Mexico, and no other family members were ill now. Both parents were field workers and the girl spent her days in a day care where no other children were known to have been ill recently.

On examination, she had a temperature of 41°C (105.5°F). She was groggy and lethargic. She was well nourished and well hydrated. She answered simple questions in inappropriate monosyllables, or by deferring to her mother. She had enlarged, moderately inflamed tonsils, but showed an entirely normal physical examination otherwise. In particular, there were no signs of meningismus, peritoneal irritation, adventitious breath sounds, cardiac murmurs, or soft tissue inflammation.

Although there were no signs of focal infection other than tonsillitis, because she appeared sick and had a very high temperature the clinician considered a serious infection to be both quite likely and very dangerous to the patient. His primary working hypothesis at this point was atypical presentation of some form of infection such as

1. meningitis
2. urinary tract infection
3. pneumonia
4. silent peritonitis and/or appendicitis
5. other deep soft tissue or bone infection
6. bacterial endocarditis
7. 1–6 above, possibly with bacteremia
8. early stage of a viral infection such as hepatitis or flulike illness

The patient was initially treated with oral Tylenol and a glass of Coca-Cola. Urinalysis, complete blood count, and lumbar puncture were done.

Within half an hour her temperature was 101°F, she was alert and oriented, her behavior was appropriate, and she offered no complaints. Her headache and abdominal pain had resolved. Complete blood count, urinalysis, and lumbar puncture were entirely normal, as were throat and blood cultures reported subsequently. All slides were reviewed personally by the lab technician and the clinician.

The response to Tylenol, the improvement in her appearance, and the negative lab work were reassuring, and greatly reduced the probability of an emergent bacterial infection. Although these possibilities were not entirely ruled out, the clinician judged that the patient could safely be treated on an outpatient basis.

Tonsillitis provided a plausible, though not satisfying, explanation of the clinical picture. She was treated with amoxicillin and regular doses of Tylenol. Because of the very high fever and acute onset, the girl and her mother were instructed to return the following day for reexamination, and to call if anything new developed in the meantime or if significant headache or abdominal pain recurred.

When seen the following day, she was afebrile, complained only of sore throat and mild back ache, and her exam was entirely normal. The clinician was reassured.

The next day she presented again with shaking, high fever, headache, and abdominal pain. Temperature was 105.5°F. She looked ill. Physical exam was otherwise normal. The same hypotheses were again entertained. In addition, the clinician noted (he had to write these hypotheses down to remember them all)

1. less common infectious diseases with recurring fever such as brucellosis and tuberculosis

2. familial fever
3. autoimmune disease
4. other metabolic or drug-related recurring fevers
5. malignancy
6. metabolic disorder such as porphyria or familial Mediterranean fever

All of these new hypotheses were relatively unfamiliar as causes of recurring fever to the clinician, who planned to review them briefly while the patient underwent a complete blood count, urinalysis, and a chest x-ray, and arrangements were made for hospital admission.

On this occasion, the girl's complete blood count was again normal. However, an alert lab technician fortuitously decided to review the smear again, and recognized misshapen and fragmented red cells characteristic of malaria.

Lessons To Be Learned

1. It is appropriate, and often necessary, to initiate treatment very early in the encounter. In this case, early treatment of the fever enabled the girl to respond appropriately to interview, and made her much easier to evaluate. The rapid drop in temperature provided a degree of reassurance that she did not have an overwhelming infection. As it turned out, symptomatic treatment was all that could be provided at the first interview.

   It is essential to recognize when you don't know. You must, nonetheless, manage the patient without a firm diagnosis.

2. It is often not possible to establish a firm or a satisfying diagnosis at the first encounter,

or even one that has a reasonable probability of being correct. The correct diagnosis may not even be in your list of hypotheses. When this happens, one may treat the "plausible" diagnosis (tonsillitis in this case) as a pathologic entity, but must remain acutely aware that the picture is incomplete and therefore remain very alert to other hypotheses. Therapeutic efforts are focused on the patient's symptoms and signs, and attention is directed to the response to therapy. In this circumstance it is essential to follow the patient very closely, and to give her access to reevaluation at any time—night or day—should the clinical picture change. If the patient's safety is in question, further investigation or an immediate consultation is in order.

3. The clinician was comfortable in sending the patient home when he was unable to establish a firm diagnosis. He focused on deciding whether or not the patient was dangerously ill (in which case she should be admitted to the hospital, and immediate consultation obtained). He decided that the girl was not critically ill, and could safely be followed closely as an outpatient. The clinician was reassured by the patient's normal complete blood count and CSF (cerebrospinal fluid), her prompt clinical response to Tylenol, and that she did not have a serious bacterial infection. Therefore he could treat the girl's apparent tonsillitis with amoxicillin, without significant risk of obscuring a serious underlying infection.

4. The diagnosis of malaria did not even occur to the clinician in the initial encounter, or

in the second, despite an unusually long list of possible conditions. You will seldom include every possible diagnosis in your list of hypotheses. However, if you cannot establish a satisfying, reasonably firm diagnosis, the correct diagnosis will usually become manifest upon time, reexamination, another opinion, or good fortune. In the meantime, your patients are very unlikely to come to harm if you focus on the pathophysiologic alterations (basic science) and direct your treatment to restoring altered physiology and biochemistry toward normal to maintain the patient's relative well-being. (This is absolutely essential. In some cases, patients may be treated for years without a specific diagnosis ever being established.)

CONTINUING WITH THE REASONING PROCESS

As you proceed in the evaluation process with the patient, you should be thinking about how you are going to manage the patient's problem: medicines, surgery, counseling, when and where? You will need to finalize these thoughts when you decide upon the best explanation for the patient's problem at the end of the encounter. Some of these treatment or management thoughts will raise questions that you need to ask the patient during the encounter. Most clinicians tend to mix these management-related questions with their hypothesis-oriented inquiry strategy. Such questions concern

Always keep your real goal—helping the patient with his or her problem—in mind.

medications the patient is taking that might conflict with proposed medication, allergies to medication, illnesses that could be provoked by treatment, readiness to come into the hospital, and so on.

Part of the overall inquiry strategy to resolve hypotheses goes beyond the history and physical examination. This is the use of laboratory tests and diagnostic procedures to provide further needed data, which will be considered in the next chapter. However, you should jot down your management and laboratory test ideas on your note pad as you go along in the encounter. You can review these when you are finished. An available note pad is a convenient extra memory for noting concerns to be followed up on later. However, do not let the note pad come between you and your patient. Use it sparingly!

9

Laboratory and Diagnostic Tests

Laboratory and diagnostic tests are additional inquiry-strategy tools for obtaining further, sometimes crucial, information, to resolve the hypotheses entertained. However, tests involve delay, cost, risk, and inconvenience for the patient. These factors require consideration of benefits and costs in your reasoning process.

SHORT-LOOP AND LONG-LOOP INFORMATION RETRIEVAL: QUICK VS. DELAYED ANSWERS

During the patient encounter, data come instantly. Ask a question, and the answer is immediately available. You can analyze the answer and ask another question. It is a *short loop*. You can pursue any course of inquiry that seems productive and then change to other inquiry strategies when the strategy being pursued is no longer productive. The same is true with a physical examination. The short response time allows great freedom to follow

History and physical are short-loop inquiry tools.

the inquiry strategy that seems most productive. When a strategy no longer seems productive, you can scan for new leads or try alternative strategies. The patient problem unfolds before the examiner in a matter of minutes.

Questions and examinations, as individual items, have little cost. The encounter, as a total package, has an identifiable cost in both time and money, but the individual questions and items of examination can be variable in depth and number without adding concerns for the overall cost. There is essentially no risk for the patient in an inquiry process that involves only history and physical. Inept questions with a disturbed or worried patient, or too many questions in a life-threatening emergency can carry a risk, but this is not a usual situation. It's important to consider the history- and physical-based inquiry as a short loop with low cost, in order to put the use of laboratory tests and diagnostic procedures into their proper perspective.

Laboratory and diagnostic tests are long-loop inquiry tools.

Laboratory tests—studies of blood, urine, spinal fluid, exhaled air, feces, or body products in general—can rarely be performed by the clinician or someone else in the immediate clinical environment so that the results of the test can be known during the patient encounter. The results of these tests are characteristically delayed from hours to days. A few tests can be performed at the time of the encounter with rapid turnaround such as blood count, hemoglobin, urine analysis, and mono spot. However, even these tests are commonly employed in a manner that produces a delay: the clinician receives the results after the patient encounter. Diagnostic procedures are more elaborate studies of the human body, such as x-rays and other imaging techniques, x-rays taken by themselves or after the introduction of a contrast medium or radioactive substance into the gut, blood vessels, joints, subarachnoid space, etc. Scans of injected radioactive materials, biopsies of various tissues of the body, magnetic resonance imaging, electroencephalograms, electrocardiograms, exercise studies, to name only a very few, are diagnostic procedures. Some may require a stay in the diagnostic laboratory or a stay in the hospital, with special types of patient preparation. Diagnostic procedures require the services of a specially trained clinician to interpret the results of the study. For our purposes, both laboratory and diagnostic procedures can be grouped together as *tests*. All tests represent a *long-loop* inquiry, and therefore represent a different strategy (see Figure 11).

COST CONSIDERATIONS IN DIAGNOSTIC TESTS

Appropriateness

There is ever-increasing concern among health insurance companies, employers, the government, and the public over the increasing expense of tests. This expense, paid for out of the patient's pocket or by third-party providers, has become a national issue. Increasing evidence indicates that tests are misused or used unnecessarily. There are numerous causes for this problem. One relates to the aims of this book: Clinicians often do not approach the patient's problem with appropriate scientific rigor, by applying the clinical-reasoning process

The misuse of tests is in large part due to sloppy or lazy thinking during the patient encounter.

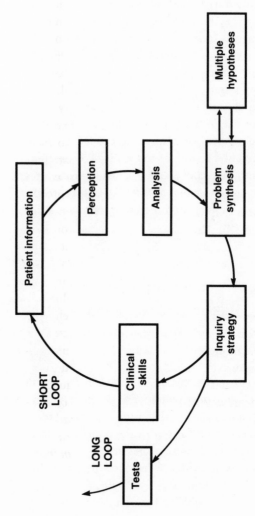

FIGURE 11. The use of diagnostic procedures and laboratory tests (called "Tests" in diagram) represent a long-loop inquiry strategy. The results are not learned by the clinician during the encounter.

carefully in the history and physical examination to resolve the problem as far as possible by the use of powerful but inexpensive clinical-reasoning tools during the history and physical examination. Instead, there is a strong tendency to rely on tests to diagnose the problem, with little thinking occurring on the clinician's part. This is an inefficient and ineffective use of investigative tools that are often expensive, time-consuming, painful, and risky. Another cause for the problem is many clinicians' lack of awareness of the actual expense, discomfort, and risks of tests, contrasted to their actual value in aiding diagnosis and treatment. *They do not have an awareness of benefits versus costs.* Many tests are employed or requested merely because they are habitually performed with certain types of patient problems, without regard for their actual value or need in the particular patient problem. Some clinicians, particularly those in postgraduate educational settings, have the feeling that they are not being scientific in their evaluation unless they order every conceivable test, a behavior often rewarded and sometimes even expected by clinical faculty. Another factor is the clinician's lack of knowledge about test specificity and sensitivity—the left side of the benefit/cost equation. *Tests ordered as a substitute for thinking, or tests ordered on the basis of unquestioned tradition, have served to escalate the cost of health care for all of us and expose countless patients to unnecessary costs and risks.*

Many clinicians are unaware of test cost, test risk, and even test value in their work with the patient.

Common Uses

Only a fraction of tests are used to establish a diagnosis. In fact, very few tests are diagnostic.

The common uses of tests are

1. *To lend some evidence for one or more hypotheses on your list.* For example, ST segment elevation on the electrocardiogram is consistent with (but certainly not diagnostic of) myocardial ischemia. An infiltrate on chest x-ray is consistent with pneumococcal pneumonia (but also consistent with several other disease processes).

2. *To assess the severity and follow the course of a disease.* For example, a very simple test—erythrocyte sedimentation rate—is a very useful indicator of the activity and severity of rheumatoid arthritis. As the disease becomes more active, the sed rate rises, as the disease either responds to treatment or spontaneously remits, the sed rate falls. A white blood cell count is very useful in assessing a patient's response to infection. Both tests are very nonspecific, however, and of no specific *diagnostic* value.

3. *To reassure either the patient or the clinician.* Increasingly, this use of laboratory tests is justified, or at least rationalized, by medicolegal anxieties. Although it is not necessarily borne out in practice, clinicians feel much more discomfort and anxiety, and perceive more legal risk, in not doing extensive testing than in doing extensive testing. They treat their anxiety by ordering additional testing that is not of clear value.

Role in Inquiry Strategy

Used appropriately, tests are powerful inquiry tools for the clinician.

Tests, like the history and physical examination, are part of the armamentarium of the clinician in inquiring about a patient's problem. They can offer unique information that can be decisive in the care of the patient when used appropriately. However, unlike the short-loop, low-cost, low-risk history and physical inquiry, tests are longer-loop, higher cost, riskier inquiries. Since the results usually are not known until after the patient encounter, and sometimes take weeks to return to the clinician, the nature of the inquiry strategy is significantly changed. On history you can ask a question, and the answer to that question will provide information that will indicate the next question you should ask. However, with tests, the serial approach could take months. A test may be ordered in which the results might then indicate a need for yet another test. This in turn will take a number of days. In such a serial or sequential manner, the inquiry strategy may take so long that the patient may have recovered or died before you know what was going on. In any inquiry strategy employing tests, the clinician has to "hedge his bets." He needs to request *all* the tests that will be essential in verifying the hypotheses remaining at the end of the encounter and all tests that are essential to decisions about the anticipated management plan. This does not mean the clinician needs to order every test in the book—just the *right* ones. This decision requires an awareness of important benefit/cost aspects of tests.

> The strategies required for long-loop inquiry involve, among other things, "hedging your bets."

Sensitivity, Specificity, and Relevance

These are important characteristics of a test that you must understand in order to use tests most effectively and economically.

1. *Sensitivity:* How well does the test detect the presence of the suspected disease process, or

> Sensitivity, specificity, and relevance are estimates of a test's value or benefit.

substantiate an entertained hypothesis? That is, how sensitive is it to the presence of the disease? How unlikely is it that this test will come out with a *falsely negative* result even if the disease is present in the patient? This measurement of sensitivity can be expressed as the percentage of patients with the disease suspected that will show a positive test result. You may have trouble finding this expressed as a fixed percentage for many of the tests you wish to use, but you must learn whether the test is very sensitive, moderately sensitive, or only somewhat better than chance in detecting the disease.

2. *Specificity:* How specific is this test for the disease process suspected? This can be formally expressed as the percentage of patients without the suspected disease who will show a negative result. This helps you consider how often the test will be *falsely positive* in patients that do not have the disease. Again, this is a figure that may not be easy to find, but you should have a ball-park idea of the test's specificity.

3. *Relevance:* Considering sensitivity and specificity, how important is the test to your working hypothesis, or to ruling out other possible hypotheses that may affect prognosis or management? Will the test really make a difference in the diagnosis and management of the patient? Relevance requires that you ask the following questions about any test that you propose:
   a. How will I manage my patient if the test shows a negative result?

b. How will I manage my patient if the test shows a positive result?

If there is no difference in the answer to these two questions, then it is hard to justify the test. If there is a difference, and the test will have an impact on the care of your patient (either through establishing the working diagnosis or the nature of the problem), is that impact worth the cost?

Benefit/Cost Ratio

These are other considerations you must entertain with every test you order to compare value against drawbacks.

Price tag: The price for the patient as well as the health-care system involved. This includes the cost of the test itself, the cost of its interpretation, the cost of time in the hospital and of the use of personnel and other materials. You must know the costs of the tests you order. Keep a reference handy.

Cost, time delay, discomfort, and risk are the negative values to be weighed against possible benefit.

Time delay: How long does it take to get the results? There are usually two time delays to be considered—the time it takes to get the test routinely and the time it takes to get the test when you order it as an emergency.

Inconvenience and/or discomfort: What is required of the patient in terms of time, travel, and preparation? What discomforts are there? Are embarrassment, waiting, medication, side effects, or *pain* involved? You should know this in intimate detail, not only to appreciate the negative aspects that may weigh against the possible benefits of the test, but to be able to *properly prepare the patient for what he or she will be facing.*

Risk: Many diagnostic procedures carry a risk, both in terms of morbidity (that is, temporary or permanent symptoms or disability that may result from the test) and in terms of mortality. These risks can vary with the patient's age and illness. Although these morbidity/mortality figures are easier to come by than those for inconvenience/discomfort, they still may not be found readily for many diagnostic procedures. *You must know if the risk of the procedure or test you are ordering is greater than the risk of the patient's illness.* Again, you should know if the risks are high (10% or more), moderate (5% or less), or minimal (less than 1%).

In summary, you have a benefit/cost ratio to carry out.

$$\frac{\text{Benefit (sensitivity + specificity + relevance)}}{\text{Cost (price + time delay + inconvenience + risk)}}$$

This ratio is an informal guide to your weighing of benefit versus costs. *It is not to be taken literally as an equation.*

10

Diagnostic Decision-Making

You cannot care for your patient unless you have an idea of what is wrong. A diagnostic decision has to be made before you treat. In most instances, all the data you would like to have to make this decision are not available, despite a detailed and effective inquiry. You have to decide what in all likelihood is wrong with the patient so that you can care for the patient even if the diagnosis is not a sure thing. You have to play the odds in favor of the patient. There is risk and responsibility in this task. Diagnostic decision-making is one of the great professional challenges in medicine.

THE DIAGNOSIS

The Most Likely Working Hypothesis: Guidelines for the Diagnostic Decision

The first decision that needs to be made before the patient encounter can end is the diagnosis (or final working hypothesis), as shown in Figure 12. The clinician must decide on the most likely work-

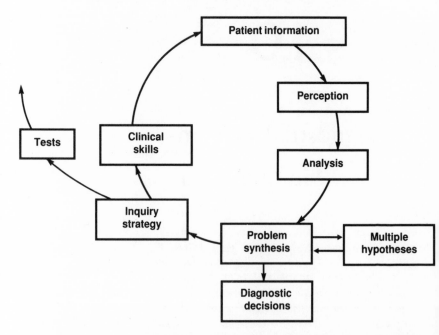

FIGURE 12. When the problem synthesis, as the result of inquiry, is seen to resemble one of the hypotheses entertained, the clinician often accepts that hypothesis as his final working hypothesis, or diagnosis. He has made a diagnostic decision. The competing hypotheses need to be kept in mind as further tests (long loops) may be required to be certain of the diagnosis and to eliminate definitely the remaining hypotheses.

Making the diagnostic decision with the evidence available.

ing hypothesis or hypotheses to explain the patient's problem. Many have pointed out that medicine is an imperfect science. There are few perfect ones. Or that the clinician has to live with ambiguity. Who doesn't? Or that decisions have to be made on insufficient data. Probably so. All of this is true. Expression of disease is variable; each patient is unique in response and style. Measureable, objective data about the functional integrity of any organ including the psyche, are limited. The clinician has to interpret an individual's symptoms, signs, and test results against calculated norms for populations in general and the accumulated wisdom in medicine concerning the manifestations of disease.

As described in Chapter 7, to arrive at this decision the clinician tries to obtain data from the patient that will allow him to develop or shape the problem synthesis to fit one of his hypotheses. This "fit" occurs if the patient is found to present enough of the expected positive and negative findings collected under the clinician's hypothesis label—enough to give the clinician the impression that the hypothesis explains the patient's problem. The fit occurs if the assumed underlying pathophysiology matches with the working hypothesis selected. A perfect fit rarely happens. This is why you will rarely see the textbook case. Some helpful textbooks will describe the frequency of certain symptoms and signs; however, *a decision has to be made*. Unlike the scientist, the clinician cannot put off making a decision to get more data or to do more research. When you face the inevitable need to make a diagnostic decision at the end of the patient encounter, the following guidelines may be helpful:

1. Is there enough evidence in your problem synthesis to decide that one of the hypotheses can be accepted as a tentative, or working, diagnosis?
2. Is there enough evidence in your problem synthesis to suggest the likely diagnosis, or working hypothesis, pending confirmation by tests, response to treatment, or information from subsequent events?
3. If two or more hypotheses still seem equally

possible, will further tests, consultations, reexaminations, or subsequent response to therapy help sort them out? In this instance, please remember *common things occur commonly.* If one of your two or more equally likely hypotheses or diagnoses occur with much less frequency in the patient population, it can usually be given a lower priority in your decision-making. If the symptoms or signs in your patient, as assembled in the problem synthesis, occur far more often in one of the hypotheses than in the others, then that hypothesis should probably receive a higher priority in your diagnostic decision-making. Don't forget that the patient population you see in a particular setting may be different than the populations in the general community. Specialty settings have the puzzling or complex patients referred to them. The bias this produces in disease likelihood or frequency must be appreciated.

4. If no discrete, sophisticated, specific, or refined diagnosis is really possible, the final working hypothesis should be *stated in more general terms,* followed by the possible but as yet unsubstantiated more refined diagnoses (which must be ruled out by subsequent tests, consultations, reexaminations, etc.). (For example, a general diagnosis of "chest pain due to the anginal syndrome; myocardial infarction and musculoskeletal pain to be ruled out," or general diagnosis of "cervical spinal cord lesion; intermedullary hemorrhage, metastases, transverse myelitis to be ruled out.")

5. If the therapies for the entertained hypotheses

are the same, or if the prognoses are essentially the same, perhaps further refinement in your diagnostic decision-making may not be immediately necessary.

6. Is it necessary to reach a diagnosis at this time, or can the diagnosis be deferred until after a period of observation? In this instance, you would carry along the problem synthesis and the collection of tentative hypotheses you have been working with. "Tincture of time" often resolves many problems in medicine.

That is the first step.

WHEN THE DIAGNOSIS IS STILL IN DOUBT

Alternative Hypotheses

There will be times when the clinician must still carefully consider alternative hypotheses. These may occur if any of the following concerns seem appropriate:

1. Are there one or more less likely hypotheses that still need to be ruled out because they represent a greater potential threat of morbidity or mortality? Does the dizzy patient with Ménière's disease actually have a cerebellopontine tumor? The tumor is less likely statistically but can produce the same clinical picture and must be recognized early to allow for effective surgical treatment. The 62-year-old man in Chapter 7 was found to have a fairly typical picture of cholecystitis, yet carci-

Consider the infrequent but dangerous condition among your hypotheses.

noma and hepatitis were a major worry and still needed to be ruled out. If one of the competing hypotheses is a potentially serious disease that can be ameliorated or reversed by timely treatment, the possibility of its presence should be assiduously pursued.

Frequent conditions appear frequently: diagnostic decisions need to be biased in the favor of the patient's future health.

2. Are there one (or more) hypotheses that, although less likely, still need to be ruled out because they are of a high incidence in the community or in that type of patient? Tuberculosis may be most likely, but in southern California be sure coccidiomycosis is not present since it is far more prevalent there and closely resembles tuberculosis clinically. A flulike illness with abdominal pain may seem benign, but in blacks it may represent sickle-cell disease, which is not benign and if present needs to be recognized and treated. An upper respiratory illness in students could be infectious mononucleosis. In army recruits, the same picture could represent the much rarer but highly fatal meningococcic meningitis. You should always be aware of the prevalence of diseases. Prevalence is always an important factor in considering possible likely alternative hypotheses in a differential diagnosis.

3. If the most obvious diagnosis is a condition that is poorly treatable or carries a poor prognosis, the clinician must make sure that *any* treatable (or less malignant) condition, although unlikely, might not be the correct diagnosis. Even though it may seem obvious that a patient has a motoneuron disease (which carries a fatal prognosis and has no treatment), the less likely or even remote pos-

sibility of cervical spondylosis needs to be considered. A pleural effusion in a patient with carcinoma would obviously suggest metastases of the carcinoma, but it might also indicate a congestive heart failure that needs to be recognized and treated. The exacerbation of malignancy could be due to malnutrition. Schizophrenia could represent toxicity from carbon monoxide, lead, or mercury.

There are an increasing number of computer software programs becoming available that will help you think of alternative hypotheses to explain your patient's problem. The computer, with its large memory of recallable data to complement your reasoning and judgment, can offer you a powerful tool. You can enter your patient data and these programs will generate alternative hypotheses for you to consider, often with information about the symptoms, signs, and expected laboratory findings with each hypothesis. You can then choose those that, in your judgment, seem possible and reasonable.

MR. HAWKINS

The cardiology consultant agrees with the clinician's assessment of Mr. Hawkins. The patient is scheduled for immediate coronary angiography to clearly define his coronary anatomy and the functional status of his myocardium, and to help the clinician make a definitive treatment decision and proceed with it.

The clinician returns to Mr. Hawkins.

The next step is to make sure that there are no other problems, possibly nonmedical, confronting the patient that may affect your patient's response to treatment, recovery, sense of well-being, attitude, or ability to return to work or achieve a gainful social role.

- psychological factors such as depression, anxiety, poor self-image
- economic factors such as debt or lack of employment
- social factors such as problems with family, friends, peers, cultural group, work environment
- handicaps or physical disabilities
- other illnesses, particularly chronic illnesses

Lastly, the clinician must be certain that there are no unexplained complaints, findings on examination, or laboratory results (present or past) that need further analysis or that need to be followed.

Tentative Diagnoses

At best, the diagnosis is a working hypothesis made in an imperfect world—but it must be made.

Students often have the false belief that in order to decide on a hypothesis as a diagnosis, all the symptoms, signs, and laboratory findings described in the textbooks are necessary. As this is rarely the case, you have to learn to make a pragmatic decision so that an appropriate course of action can be taken with your patient. So do it—*make a diagnosis*. No diagnosis should ever be thought of as cast in bronze. It is always a working hypothesis or diagnosis. Your decision always represents the best working hypothesis possible at the time, subject to change pending new information. You must make a decision and have appropriate confidence in that decision. Your subsequent work with the patient should reflect this confidence. In medicine it is no sin to admit that your diagnosis is tentative. It *is* a sin to make your diagnosis more refined than the data really allow. This takes a delicate balance of decision-making before all the evidence is in, yet being totally honest when a refined decision is clearly not warranted. Making too refined a diagnosis can close your mind to other possibilities. Making too vague a diagnosis may forestall appropriate management. This is a thinking skill to be exercised again and again.

> The diagnosis must not be more specific than the data allow.

You must commit yourself in writing at the end of the encounter so that you can learn by your errors, and modify your subsequent performance. If you do not commit yourself, and the patient turns out differently than you expected, you will have a tendency to say later, "Oh, yeah, I thought of that at the time—I just didn't want to say so." The "retrospectroscope" is always clouded by the passage of time. At the end of the encounter write down your diagnostic decisions *and why you made them*.

> Keep a record of your decisions and your reasons; by doing so, you begin a powerful chain of learning sequences.

You must practice being comfortable making decisions on inadequate or conflicting data, to take calculated risks in the interest of helping your patient when the science of medicine cannot resolve the problem.

THE DIAGNOSIS IS A GUIDE TO INQUIRY: THE PROBLEM SYNTHESIS

Remember that the problem synthesis is *really* your patient's problem. The diagnostic decision you made provides a label to guide further investi-

> The diagnosis is of no value without the problem synthesis; they complement each other.

Be attentive to data that do not fit your diagnoses.

gation, to select appropriate treatment, and to classify the patient's problem for record-keeping and statistical purposes. *Always* be aware of the aspects of your patient that may not fit the chosen diagnosis well, as these exceptions may explain further findings as you treat and follow the patient. Remaining aware of the exceptions will prevent you from accepting the diagnosis you choose as cast in bronze and will open your eyes to poor responses to treatment, unusual test results, or new symptoms. These observations will alert you to the need to reconsider your diagnosis. (It could even lead to your uncovering a new diagnostic entity.)

Your patient synthesis guides your management of and relationship to the patient, and invites the patient's active involvement. It is useful to think of the patient's problem (and your problem synthesis) as three concentric spheres. In the center is the disease, (usually the diagnosis, the altered molecular biology). Part of your treatment is directed toward this hard pathology. There may or may not be specific treatments for the pathologic process. The disease is contained within the patient's illness. The illness is also composed of the patient's response to the disease, how he feels, how he perceives it, what he understands about it and how it affects his ability to function physically and socially in his work and in looking after himself.

The patient's illness is contained within his life situation. (This outer circle also comprises the patient's environment and the reciprocal effects of his family members and significant others, his work situation, and his community.)

Each of these spheres are included in a fully developed patient synthesis. Your management and the patient's participation in that management are directed toward the patient as a person, as a member of a society, and as a member of a family, as well as toward the pathologic disease process.

MR. HAWKINS

The clinician asks Mr. Hawkins

"What do you understand about what is happening to you, and what are your concerns so far?"

This question must be phrased carefully. If you ask a patient "What do you think is wrong with you?" you will very often get the response, "That is why I'm here," or "That is your job to find out."

Mr. Hawkins responds, "I think I am having a heart attack. It sure seems like what my father and my brother had. Am I going to do okay? What should I tell my wife? Should we call our sons? Can you do something to control this?"

The clinician explains her understanding of the problem to the patient in very straightforward terms.

"Yes, you appear to be having a heart attack. This is caused by inadequate blood supply to your heart muscle resulting from obstruction or blockage of one or more of the arteries that supply your heart muscle. Your heart seems to be functioning well as a pump at this point, and you have not developed any complications so far. With treatment your outlook is pretty good. With you in the hospital, if complications develop, we can treat them immediately.

"At this point, since your pain only started two hours ago, you probably have suffered very little permanent injury to your cardiac muscle. There are two courses we can take. We can watch you in the coronary care unit and give you medication to relieve your pain, in which case you will have some permanent damage to your heart muscle. Exactly how much we can't predict, but otherwise you should make a good recovery. Alternatively, we can treat you aggressively by doing an angiogram—special x-rays where we inject a dye that shows up on x-ray directly into your heart's arteries through a thin plastic catheter that we put into your artery in your groin. This will allow us to see exactly where the blockage is and decide how to treat it. Depending on the nature of the blockage, we can treat it either by opening it up with a balloon on the catheter, or with a chemical that dissolves clots—or you may require surgery. I very strongly encourage you to take the latter course because the end result will very likely be better. You may recover, with little or no damage to your heart muscle. In the long run, of course, we will have to do some things to prevent you from having a future heart attack, including your quitting smoking, and taking up regular exercise. But we will talk about that later. Do you understand what I have told you so far? What questions do you have?"

Mr. and Mrs. Hawkins and the clinician discuss the management alternatives, risks and costs, and prognosis in more detail.

The clinician left the couple alone for a few minutes before asking them to agree to her advised plan, or to make another decision.

PATIENT EDUCATION

The clinician has now undertaken patient education. As you can see, it is an important part of the treatment. It is covered in more detail in Chapter 13.

11

Therapeutic Decision-Making

The therapeutic decision is the whole purpose of your encounter with the patient. Are you able to cure the patient, alleviate his or her symptoms, improve on the natural course of the illness, minimize or avoid complications? Is your treatment worth the cost and potential risk or possible discomfort? Again, choices have to be made sensitive to these benefit/cost factors, the patient's needs, and his or her value system. The choices often have to be made on limited data.

DESIGNING THE THERAPEUTIC PROGRAM

Understanding the Problem

Herbert Simon sees the clinician's task as one of "design."

Herbert Simon, well known for his research and writing in the field of human problem-solving, described the task of the professional as one of design. He defined *design* as devising "courses of action aimed at changing existing situations into preferred ones" [*The Sciences of the Artificial*, (Cambridge,

Mass: M.I.T. Press, 1970, p. 55)]. This is how
to view the task of the clinician as a health professional: to devise a course of action aimed at changing a patient's existing unacceptable situation into
a preferred one. The change must be a cure, a
relief of pain, an improvement in health status, a
prevention of impending illness or complication,
or a reduction of distress or concern, depending
upon the patient's objectives and your objectives.
As has been stated many times before, in order
to help the patient the clinician must inquire. The
information the clinician needs to design the right
treatment is not laid out in the initial encounter.
With obvious problems (or problems in which the
method of evaluation is cut and dried), evaluation
may not play a large role, then design becomes
the principle activity.

Cut-and-dried approaches to evaluations are
usually seen with experts working with common
problems in the area of their specialty. The novice
has the challenge of carefully evaluating the patient
problem until it becomes familiar, and he or she
knows the strategies to evaluate the cause and treatment rapidly. In all instances, however, the clinician must have a sufficient initial diagnostic understanding of the problem to design appropriate
management or treatment.

Treatment, the Ultimate Goal

The design perspective puts evaluation in the
correct relationship to treatment. Eight chapters
have been spent on patient evaluation. You could
easily think that diagnosis is the big endeavor in
medicine—an end in itself. Careful, scientific evaluation of the patient is only a *means of choosing*

Treatment is the goal of
the clinician—patient
encounter, not
diagnosis.

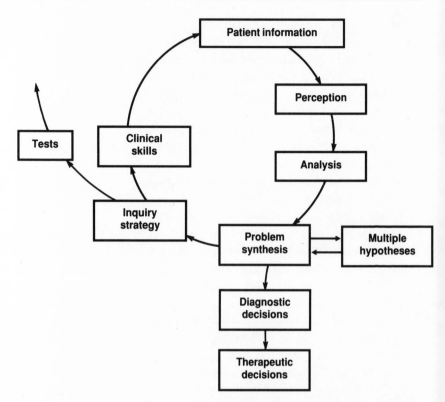

FIGURE 13. Once the diagnosis or final working hypothesis has been chosen (sometimes before) the clinician also decides on the therapeutic (or management) plan.

the appropriate treatment. The clinician's most important decision is the management plan (the therapeutic decisions demonstrated in Figure 13). Part of this decision is the selection of appropriate long-loop inquiries—the tests needed to evaluate the patient further or to select the best treatment.

TREATMENT DECISIONS IN THE PATIENT ENCOUNTER

As mentioned in the previous chapter, clinicians are often observed to consider treatment approaches early in the encounter while they are evaluating the patient. As symptoms emerge, they think of how they may have to treat them. Many times the treatment of the symptom may be the same for different hypotheses, as the pathophysiological mechanisms producing the symptoms are the same for each. At this early stage, the clinician may consider alternative approaches to treatment: medicine as opposed to surgery, medicine as opposed to physical therapy, particular classes of pharmaceutical agents, and so forth. During inquiry of the patient to diagnose the patient's problems the clinician frequently asks questions related to treatment ideas that he may be entertaining interdigitated with questions relevant to his diagnostic hypotheses. Such questions, described before, may refer to prior response to medication, intolerance to drugs, drug allergies, and so on.

Diagnostic ideas, treatment ideas, and hypotheses are often entertained in a simultaneous or intertwined fashion during the patient workup, leading to the eventual diagnostic and therapeutic decisions.

EXAMPLE

Recall the 4-year-old girl with acute lower abdominal pain who was initially seen in Chapter 4. Early in the encounter with this patient the clinician needed to determine whether the girl required

1. observation and symptomatic treatment only
2. medical treatment, fluids, electrolytes, and antibiotics
3. surgical treatment

These management hypotheses help suggest other questions. For example, if there were signs indicating dehydration, toxicity, or high temperature, more aggressive treatment would be warranted. If signs of peritoneal irritation were present, surgical intervention would be likely.

THE DIAGNOSTIC THERAPEUTIC TRIAL

If the treatment works, your diagnostic decision is supported.

Many interventions can be both diagnostic and therapeutic. For example, when a clinician has difficulty differentiating between causes of visceral chest pain, he may give the patient nitroglycerin. If the pain is relieved, that points toward esophageal spasm or myocardial ischemia. He may then give the patient a cocktail of liquid antacid, an anticholinergic and antispasmodic, and a viscous local anesthetic. If this cocktail relieves the pain, it provides fairly strong evidence pointing toward esophageal pain.

Treatment can be therapeutic and can continue the diagnostic process as well.

In the case of a patient presenting with symptoms strongly suggestive of acid peptic disease, it is usual to initiate treatment without establishing a diagnosis. If the initial treatment of H2 histamine receptor blockers and/or antacid relieves the patient's symptoms, this response provides very strong evidence in support of the acid peptic disease hypothesis. Only if the patient does not respond will many clinicians proceed with a further diagnostic workup.

Mr. Hawkins

The clinician's management objectives for Mr. Hawkins are

1. immediate relief of pain
2. myocardial salvage by reestablishing perfusion
3. prevention, or recognition and treatment, of complications
4. prevention of recurrence by
   a. continuing medical therapies
   b. altering risk factors through patient education, change in behavior, and medical treatment
5. further refinement of the problem synthesis and diagnosis
6. further definition and institution of management for other medical problems such as gout and diabetes through patient education and behavioral change.

Note that the patient's response to the treatment plan will also provide further diagnostic information.

Decisions Early in the Patient Encounter

When Is Therapy Actually Considered?

Here is another case we have considered previously: a 62-year-old man with acute upper abdominal pain.

In this instance the clinician will consider treatment to relieve pain early in the encounter. The type of analgesia used will depend upon the most likely hypothesis in the clinician's mind at the time. The patient's response to the specific analgesic may also help to eliminate or strengthen one or more hypothesis: rapid relief of the pain with nitroglycerin would suggest atypical angina or esophagitis; relief with an antacid would support peptic ulcer; exacerbation of the pain on drinking the antacid might make pancreatitis more likely.

When a clinician sees a problem such as a 6-month-old baby with a temperature of 40.5°C, he will very often decide to treat the fever before much more history and physical are carried out. The clinician does this because an irritable, lethargic child is harder to evaluate and because a child with a high temperature is at greater risk for seizure. A child whose fever does not respond readily to treatment is more likely to have a *serious* illness. If the child is vomiting, the route to administer medication needs to be considered.

It is confusing to try to separate the intent a clinician's questions by whether they relate primarily to diagnosis or treatment concerns or both. However, by the end of the inquiry for the best diagnostic decision or working hypothesis, the clinician usually has accumulated a number of ideas about treatment as well. He also has formed ideas about where treatment and further investigations should occur (such as at home, in the office, or in the hospital).

As treatment ideas occur to you during the history and physical, write them down.

Even though you may have developed a list of tests and managements you plan to carry out with a patient by the time a diagnostic decision is made, you may need to consider these options more formally towards the end of the inquiry (Figure 13).

Your ultimate treatment decision may require other tests such as blood levels of drugs and indicators of potential side effects or complications. Again, this is what the note pad is for. Hopefully, during the encounter you have written down on your note pad the treatment ideas you might wish to review. As mentioned earlier, one study on the clinician's reasoning process has suggested that most of the data necessary to come to a diagnostic conclusion is obtained before the encounter is half over; treatment decisions may have already been identified.

CONTINUING THE PATIENT ENCOUNTER

Besides treatment decisions, the clinician continues the encounter for a variety of reasons that need to be recognized. He often acquires more data to gain confidence in his final working hypotheses or diagnosis. Often he does this by repeating questions or examinations, reviewing the history as he understands it with the patient, scanning for other symptoms he might have missed, and asking about other things that might be true if his diagnostic decision is correct—again testing alternate hypotheses. The clinician also continues the encounter in order to have time to establish better rapport, gain a better understanding of the patient, prepare the patient for the diagnosis or treatment decisions, and encourage compliance.

The clinician has usually obtained all the information he needs to come to a diagnostic conclusion before the patient encounter is half over. The rest of the time is devoted to review, rapport, education, etc.

MR. HAWKINS

The clinician spent a few more minutes with Mr. Hawkins and his wife to ensure that they understood and were in agreement with the intervention plan, and to consolidate rapport. She wanted to be sure that Mr. and Mrs. Hawkins were adequately informed about the need for intervention, the risks, the outlook, and the long-term goals and plans.

FINALIZING THE THERAPEUTIC DECISION: CONSIDERATIONS IN IMPLEMENTING THERAPY

Benefit-cost decisions are an essential part of therapeutic decision-making.

To finalize his treatment decision, the clinician may attempt to narrow down possible alternatives in treatment by further questions about the patient's preferences for treatment, ability to take medication, and so on.

The benefit side of the treatment equation.

Treatment decisions should also be based on a benefit/cost analysis not unlike that used in considering tests. In your treatment decisions the following questions might be helpful for review:

1. *What is your treatment objective?* Is it to cure the patient, correct the underlying pathophysiological disorder, relieve symptoms, prevent complications, or what? These are often hard distinctions to make, but you should try. There are other reasons for treatment: prolonging life, assuring a patient that something is being done, or (don't laugh) assuring yourself that you are doing something. All of these objectives are acceptable so long as you realize what you are doing and why.

If you don't know your treatment objectives, you'll never know if your treatment was effective.

2. *How effective is the treatment for the purpose for which you are employing it?* How effective is it in correcting the pathophysiological mechanism of the disease process? How effective is it in preventing complications, relieving symptoms, and so on. What experience or knowledge has been accumulated about your treatment? Is your knowledge of its effectiveness based on a case you heard about, a drug advertisement, comments by a colleague, a journal article, the last case you tried it on, or what? If it is based on a journal article, drug advertisement, or colleague recommendation, were the recommendations based on a study? And, if so, what kind of study? Did the study involve a handful of patients or a large series? Were the patients randomly selected? Was a double-blind protocol used? What were the criteria for treatment? What were the criteria for improvement in those patients? Was a control group used? Some standard treatments, well accepted over the years, may not require this concern, but new ones certainly do.

Benefit/Cost and Benefit/Risk Ratios

The lack of knowledge you have in answering both questions in the preceding section cannot preclude your making treatment decisions, but such knowledge helps you make better decisions. For example, if there are several alternative treatments, you should probably use the one with a proven track record instead of the experimental treatment, the one that is poorly established, or the one in which patient experience has not sufficiently established effectiveness or side effects. If you have a patient who cannot tolerate or will not respond to the accepted treatments, and his condition is one in which some form of treatment is advisable because of progressive discomfort or disability, then you have a better reason for deciding on a new or less tried approach. But do it with your eyes open. In the last-ditch stand with a deteriorating patient, any good idea may warrant use. However, be certain the treatment does not aggravate the condition. In between is a whole spectrum of choices. The previous questions relate to the possible benefit of treatment. Now you need to contrast this with cost factors in the treatment as follows:

The cost side of the treatment equation.

1. *What is the expense?*
2. *What is the inconvenience or discomfort associated with the treatment?* (Pills to be taken frequently, repeated injections, treatments in clinic or office represent inconveniences and discomforts.)
3. *What risks or side effects are there?* Will the treatment produce distressing symptoms that may interfere with work, study, or life in general? What are the morbidity and mortality statistics of your treatment? Are there adverse effects on blood, heart, skin, liver, or other systems?
4. *What is the likelihood the patient will understand or comply with your treatment program?* Is there an educational or attitudinal

problem that may inhibit the effectiveness of your plan with this patient?

The Patient's Role

In benefit/cost decisions you must not only consider the disease you are treating, but also the patient. What are the patient's beliefs, values, desires, or objectives in treatment? Perhaps the patient is more willing than you might assume to live with the risk or discomforts of his or her problem. The patient may have cultural or learned dislikes for certain types of treatment. In most instances, the patient must be aware of your confidence in your diagnoses, and in the benefit/cost factors as you see them in the tests and treatments that are planned. Although this book is not aimed at covering the skills of patient education, such skills are important not only in giving the patient confidence in you as a clinician, but in allowing you to get all the information necessary to make the best decisions.

In your treatment decision, be certain you have considered all of the patient's problems or potential problems, whether they be psychological, social, economic, or whatever. Management of these problems may be an important factor in maximizing the benefit of your overall treatment program for the patient's problem. For example, in seizure patients it is frequently important to provide psychotherapeutic counseling along with anticonvulsant medication to achieve a lasting response in seizure control. In a similar manner, medical or surgical treatment will not be as successful as it might be if the patient is continuing under emotional or situational distress.

> You are not treating the patient's organ system or the patient's disease. You are treating the patient.

The Natural History of the Disease with and without Therapy

Be sure to ask yourself if your proposed treatment offers a better outcome than no treatment.

It cannot be stressed enough that you should be aware of the *expected natural course of the disease you are treating* considering the severity or present stage of the disease as manifested in your particular patient. The likelihood of progress, complications, future attacks, new symptoms, disabilities, or even death should be known for the patient's age, sex, and overall health. You must be certain that your chosen treatment plan offers *a better outcome than no treatment*. If it does offer better outcome, is it of sufficient quality to compensate for the cost, discomfort or risk.

Mr. Hawkins

Mr. Hawkins was taken to the cardiac cath lab. He was found to have a proximal complete occlusion of the left anterior descending coronary artery, and a 70% narrowing of the proximal circumflex. Both lesions were dilated with balloon angioplasty. His convalescence in the hospital was uneventful. Prior to discharge, he had a normal submaximal exercise stress test and thallium scan, and an echocardiogram demonstrating normal (60%) left ventricular ejection fraction.

With many complex patient problems, and in areas where there are a variety of alternative treatments all with varying degrees of benefits and risks, the evolving science of decision analysis can be of great benefit to clinicians.

12

Patient Education

Your treatment plan is not complete until you have designed an individualized patient education plan. The overall goals of patient education are

1. To ensure compliance. *That is, to provide the patient with enough knowledge and understanding of his problems, of the consequences, and of the expected effects and results of treatment, to enable him to understand and follow instructions and advice, and to recognize when he is satisfactorily performing the responsibilities given to him.*
2. To enable the patient to take appropriate, logical and reasoned actions in dealing with his problems.
3. To enhance healthy behavior. *This involves enabling the patient to modify his behaviors relative to a medical problem.*

DESIGNING THE PATIENT EDUCATION PLAN

The success of your treatment plan for the patient depends a great deal upon the patient. To effectively implement the therapeutic plans you

You must "activate" the patient as an informed and willing participant in your treatment plan.

have designed, you must be able to enlist the active, willing, and informed participation of the patient. To achieve this you must consider an education plan for your patient to complement your management or treatment plan.

Patient education is an essential component of virtually every patient encounter. It is often the most important, and sometimes the only, therapeutic tool you will use to enable a patient to deal with a problem. The effectiveness of every other therapeutic intervention (except in anesthetized or comatose patients) depends to a greater or lesser extent on the patient's informed compliance with treatment. The better the patient understands the need for treatment, the goals, the expected results, and the possible side effects, the more likely he will be to undergo and follow through with treatment. Seeing patients learn to manage, and sometimes resolve, their health problems is one of the most rewarding experiences of practice.

Patient compliance is essential to effective treatment.

Assessing the Patient's Educational Readiness

First you must assess "where the patient is at" regarding health-related knowledge and aptitude.

The first step in designing a patient education plan is to assess the patient's level of knowledge, ability to understand, and attitudes relevant to his health problem and about health in general. You have to individualize each patient's education, starting from *where the patient is at*.

By anticipating this need for an education plan during your history and physical, you can begin to assess where the patient is in his understanding of his problems, his ability to learn more about them, and his attitudes toward health care, medications, and treatment in general. This information should allow you to assess fairly accurately the patient's potential for working with you in managing his problem.

Actually, many of your questions can address diagnosis, treatment, and education at once. For example, you may use such questions as "What do you understand your problem to be?," "How is it affecting you?," "Why did you come in with this problem at this time?," or "What are you particularly concerned about?"

The questions you should be asking yourself are "How willing and able is the patient to actively participate in managing his problems?," "What needs to be done to facilitate this behavior?," "What is the best way to enlist the active and effective participation of the patient in changing an existing, unacceptable health situation into a preferred one?"

Planning for the Patient to Assume Long-Term Responsibility

As stated in the preceding chapter, your objective in the encounter with the patient is to assess the patient's needs and design an appropriate management plan. That management plan includes patient education. Although you will retain responsibility for executing some of these plans (prescribing medications, performing operative procedures, ordering follow-up investigations, advising the patient), most of the responsibility for the patient's long-term progress and well-being, and for the performance of many management tasks, must be as-

Complete treatment design includes an educational plan.

sumed by the patient. Your educational plan should enable the patient to assume this responsibility and effectively participate in his own management. The care of the patient is a team approach between you and the patient.

What must the patient know to comply with treatment?

Certainly the first question should cover information the patient needs to know to comply with the treatment, and to follow instructions accurately and effectively concerning medication and other treatments. Initially, the patient's management will be under your close supervision and direction, but eventually he should be able to take appropriate rational actions independently. Therefore you should also consider what the patient needs to know in order to make rational independent decisions about his care and management when he will not be under your close supervision.

How much responsibility can the patient take?

Emphasizing Patient Education Early in the Encounter

Patient education begins when you begin to take the history.

Patient education should start early in the patient encounter. You will find many opportunities during history and physical to ask questions that will cause the patient to think about the causes of his symptoms and that may enable him to consider changing his behavior—questions that sound like simple requests for information. For example, you might ask a patient with possible acid peptic disease, questions such as "Does aspirin bother your stomach?," "Do you get pain when you drink alcohol?," "How do you feel after a particularly large meal?," knowing that you will later instruct the patient to avoid alcohol, aspirin, large meals, and any foods that he finds bother his stomach.

Making the Patient Aware of Possible Complications

The next thing you must consider are symptoms that could suggest potential complications of the patient's illness or its treatment—symptoms that the patient may have to recognize and take appropriate actions such as calling you, stopping a certain medication, or changing a dosage. This can also be addressed during the history and physical examination. Suppose you ask "Have your stools ever been black?" The patient answers, "Yes, I had diarrhea two months ago, and had several very black, very tarry bowel movements." Your reply can have an educational slant: "That may mean that your ulcer was bleeding. If that ever happens again, you must call or come in and see me immediately, or, if I am not available, go to the emergency room."

Discussing Reasons for Medications With the Patient

To help the patient remember the appropriate times to take his medication, you can take opportunities during the history to help him understand the rationale behind the dosing schedule: "This medication, Cimetidine, stops your stomach from producing acid. For it to work effectively, you must take it before your stomach is stimulated to produce acid, that is, before you eat. Therefore, take one tablet half an hour before every meal. In addition, when your stomach is empty for a long period, acid has the most opportunity to damage it. Therefore, you will also take a tablet before you go to bed at night, because it is during the night that your stomach is without food for the longest period of time and most vulnerable to the acid." This provides education at the most effective time, when it is most relevant to the patient. As you can see, patient education should not be restricted to a session at the end of the encounter, but, as said before, must be woven into the history and physical. Therefore, as symptoms and signs emerge during your evaluation of the patient, you should consider what the patient must learn to understand his illness, manage symptoms and signs, monitor the course of his illness, recognize complications, and feel in control. Again, the intent of each question may be multiple—to address diagnostic or treatment concerns, to assess patient understanding and learning needs, and to educate the patient.

Clinical questions have multiple purposes.

Individualizing Patient Education

Increased understanding enables the patient to take increased responsibility.

Patient education must be carefully individualized. The ability of each individual to take part in management decisions and in self-care varies tremendously with his physical, intellectual and emotional attributes. For example, if a patient *understands* the principles of diabetic management, that patient is much more likely to manage his diet and treatment effectively and make rational decisions in his care than one who has to rely on an endless set of rules. Increasing a patient's understanding and participation in management enables him to live an increasingly normal life. A patient's ability to understand and to learn may be limited at first, and little may be accomplished in your first sessions. However, education should be looked upon as a continuous activity. As you work together over months and years, the patient's capacity for understanding will grow.

As an example of a chronic and complex illness: one goal in the management of diabetics will be to eventually transfer as much responsibility, authority, and ability for management to the patient as possible. The physician-patient relationship becomes a partnership in which the physician's role is to teach, provide technical expertise and information, and—to a greater or lesser extent—share the responsibility for making decisions. This partnership enhances control of the disease, increases patient satisfaction and sense of well-being, and may beneficially affect the long-term prognosis.

Continuing care is a partnership.

On the other hand, an acutely ill patient with pneumonia who requires intubation and respirator support can take a less active part in the management of his problem; he should, none the less, be informed as fully as possible. Your role may be paternal, as with a child or an adolescent: your guidance may be firmer, and you may shoulder a greater share of responsibility for decision-making.

A patient who is very compromised, such as a comatose patient, is unable to either understand or participate in his care. Your relationship is as to an infant. You assume full responsibility for the patient's well-being and for making treatment decisions.

Mr. Hawkins

Mr. Hawkins's postangioplasty course in the hospital was uncomplicated. The day following angioplasty, the clinician met with Mr. and Mrs. Hawkins and briefly outlined a long-term *treatment* and *education* plan, which included

1. lipid status and glucose tolerance assessment
2. weight-loss program
3. smoking-cessation program
4. graduated aerobic exercise program
5. a graduated convalescence program, with expected return to work in 4 to 6 weeks
6. reduced alcohol-consumption
7. prescription for one coated aspirin a day
8. prescriptions for other cardiac medications if and when indicated
9. blood pressure control
10. other actions to educate the patient about cardiac disease and its management, prognosis, and possible future complications (including enrollment in the hospital's cardiac rehabilitation and education program)

Avoid information overload.

Practical, concrete suggestions help to integrate changes into the patient's life.

The clinician indicated that they would discuss details and make specific plans while Mr. Hawkins remained in the hospital.

Over the next several days, Mr. Hawkins and his wife met with a nutritionist who instructed them in an 1800-calorie, high-fiber American Heart Association diet. They were both advised to follow the same diet because it would be practical to do so and they could motivate one another (and because it is generally the most appropriate diet for healthy people). They were instructed in the rationale for the diet and what it was expected to achieve. They were visited by an exercise physiologist who discussed Mr. Hawkins's graduated exercise program with them, and encouraged the participation of his wife and their adult sons.

Mr. Hawkins's lipid profile and glucose tolerance were found to be normal.

The clinician encouraged both Mr. and Mrs. Hawkins to quit smoking. She provided them with literature on quitting smoking and gave them specific suggestions on how to do it. She particularly encouraged them to work on smoking cessation, exercise, and diet together, as the mutual support would make it more practical for them and increase the probability that they would succeed. For the longer term, the clinician advised Mr. Hawkins to take up regular exercise that he could enjoy with his wife and/or their sons, because of the greater likelihood of successfully pursuing a social—as opposed to a solitary—program.

The clinician carefully outlined the nature of Mr. Hawkins's problems, their causes, their natural history, the prognosis—and the effect that risk-factor intervention might have on the prognosis. She carefully summarized and reiterated the benefits of secondary prevention and life-style modification. She also advised Mr. Hawkins about the risks and benefits of medications.

Upon discharge from the hospital, Mr. Hawkins was enrolled in a cardiac patients' education and support group.

Other Points to Consider in a Patient Education Plan

In designing your educational plan for your patient you need to ask yourself these questions.

1. What are your patient education objectives?
2. How compliant is the patient likely to become?
3. How effectively can the patient learn to follow instructions?
4. How much responsibility can the patient take if adequately informed?
5. What must the patient understand to be able to take rational action in participating in management?

Sometimes patient education will be the only therapeutic tool you use to enable the patient to fully understand his problem and learn to effectively deal with it himself. A flulike illness often requires no medication or professional treatment, but can be effectively managed by a patient who understands what to expect from the illness and how to treat the symptoms at home. A child with chickenpox or mumps may be effectively cared for at home once you have taught the parents how to assess the child's needs; how to treat the pain, itch, and other symptoms; how to control the fever and other signs; and how to recognize complications that require a clinician's intervention (such as secondary infection of the open skin lesions of chickenpox).

Minor illness may require only patient education.

APPROACHES TO PATIENT EDUCATION

You will need to use a variety of approaches to accomplish your educational plan, especially when you are dealing with a complex health problem where the patient's participation is essential. The three essential principles in applying your educational plan follow:

Simplicity: Be certain you explain things as simply as possible and in terms that the patient understands. Avoid using medical terms unless they are common. Keep your terminology appropriate to the patient's level of education and language ability. However, be sure you do not engender hostility by talking down to a patient who is capable of understanding a more sophisticated terminology. This is why it is essential for you to assess the patient's knowledge and ability to understand at the outset of the encounter.

Keep it simple.

Individualize your approach.

Repetition: Oral instructions will not be adequate unless reinforced by oral repetition and through nonverbal approaches. Use mimicry, gestures, visual demonstrations, printed material, or iteration by someone else. Anything difficult to understand or difficult to accomplish requires multiple methods of instruction.

Use multiple methods to get a point across.

Motivation: Anything that you can do to enable your patient to change his or her attitudes and behaviors will enhance the success of your efforts. Motivation will be discussed in more detail later in the chapter.

How can you motivate the patient?

TECHNIQUES FOR PATIENT EDUCATION

Oral Instructions

Avoid information overload.

Oral instructions are the most common form of patient education. As you give oral instructions, you must ask the patient to repeat in some manner what you have said to be sure he understands. Try to organize your instructions clearly, and do not provide more instruction than is really necessary. Be sure you have not given the patient more than he can digest at any one visit.

Written Instructions

Use multiple methods.

If you have complex instructions, or are faced with a patient who may have difficulty remembering, it can be very helpful to write your instructions on a note pad as you describe them orally. For extensive instructions, printed handouts are helpful. However, handouts by themselves, without your input and orientation, are ineffective. You must review the handouts with the patient if they are to be understood.

Demonstrations

Demonstrations can be very effective. You can be certain that a patient understands by having him perform a procedure after you demonstrate.

Group Classes

Group classes can be helpful for the transmission of information, but they require active participation by patients if any understanding or skill is to be gained.

Peer-Group Discussions

Peer-group sessions are extremely helpful, and provide invaluable peer reinforcement. Peers will often discuss problems they are embarrassed to bring up with a clinician. Patients profit a great deal from sharing problems and experiences. A patient can often see traits in other people that he is unable to immediately recognize in himself, or is unable to accept when confronted directly in a patient encounter. Unless you have group skills, it might be best to determine if there are good organizations in your town or trained people in your medical setting who offer group classes suited to your patient.

Behavior Modification

Behavior modification can be particularly helpful with interpersonal problems and life-style related difficulties such as obesity and addiction. However, behavior modification requires a good deal of skill and organization on the part of the therapist, and is very time consuming.

All the educational intervention in the world will be of little effect if you cannot change behaviors or attitudes that will work against the patient complying with your treatment. Behaviors and attitudes are often entrenched, and not readily modified by knowledge, understanding, or reason.

Behaviors and attitudes are not always rational.

Compliance will be a concern with a patient whose attitudes work against your plan or whose motivation for treatment is poor. The big question you face is whether the patient's behaviors and attitudes can be changed in a way that will have a positive impact on his compliance with your treatment plans. Can the patient be motivated to change his behaviors and attitudes? Behavior modification may be indicated if you have determined that the patient's behavior is part of the health problem or a potential roadblock to treatment. Although behavior modification can have an effect on rational behavior, it is more often useful in altering nonrational, unconscious, and automatic behaviors.

The patient must be *motivated* to change.

Behavior modification involves motivating the patient toward desirable behaviors by increasing the rewards of those behaviors, and decreasing the costs. Or, conversely, the patient's motivation toward undesirable behaviors can be decreased by reducing the rewards, and increasing the costs, of the undesirable behaviors.

Rewards can include increased self-esteem, the satisfaction of having learned or accomplished something, the satiation of thirst or hunger, the euphoria of tobacco or drugs, sexual satisfaction, money, prestige, and many other intrinsic or extrinsic factors.

Costs can include physical effort, mental effort required to learn something or complete an intellectual task, discomfort such as a craving for tobacco or food, physical or emotional pain, enduring risks such as the risk of falling or of being mugged taken by a frail elderly person going shopping, fatigue, the disapproval of others, peer pressure, financial costs, and so on.

When rewards exceed costs, the patient is motivated.

In manipulating this reward/cost relationship, one attempt's to modify the behavior itself, its causes, and its consequences, so as to increase the rewards of a desired behavior and decrease the costs of that behavior. On the other hand, one tries to decrease the rewards and increase the costs of undesirable or unhealthy behavior, thereby decreasing motivation and making the behavior less likely.

As an example, let us say your patient is a smoker. Behavior modification depends upon recognizing the rewards and costs of smoking and the rewards and costs of not smoking. This allows you to understand what makes your patient smoke, what makes it difficult for him to quit, and how you can help. "Of all the things you can do to help your ulcer heal, the most important is quitting smoking." (*Long-term positive consequence of desired behavior: recovery.*) "With the relatively effective treatments for ulcers that we have now, surgery is almost never necessary for either unremitting symptoms or for bleeding, except in people who continue to smoke." (*Long-term negative consequence of undesired behavior: possibility of surgery.*) (Long-term consequences, however, are not very effective motivators compared to short-term consequences.) "There are a number of things that you can do that will help you to cut down and eventually quit smoking. First of all, I will instruct you in deep-breathing exercises. This will reduce some of the nervousness that makes you smoke more." (*Modification of antecedent cause: nervousness.*): "Next, arrange to go to the office earlier—or on Saturdays—when you are relatively relaxed, so that you can do some of your work in quiet. This will reduce the stress that makes you smoke so much." (*Reduction of antecedent: stress.*)

Make practical, concrete suggestions for change.

"When you stop for a coffee break, have a bit of something to eat—an apple or an orange—instead of coffee. This will provide you with a substitute in the form of relatively nonfattening food, instead of a cigarette. Reducing your coffee consumption will reduce some of the nervousness that leads you to smoke." (*Modification of antecedents: replacement of cigarette and associated coffee with something else.*) (When a patient has something taken away, it is essential that it be replaced in some form.) "When you feel like smoking, find something else to do; get up and get a drink of water, go and talk to someone briefly, chew gum, or—when you are not at work—take some exercise." (*Modification of behaviors by substituting desirable for undesirable actions—particularly ones incompatible with smoking, such as jogging.*) "Every time you have a cigarette, make a mark on the back of the pack. At the end of the day, add up the number that you smoke. This will enable you to cut out about a third of your cigarettes." (*Change in behavior. Keeping count makes behavior more conscious, and therefore more subject to rational control. It also provides short-term goals, in terms of number of cigarettes each day.*) "When you are at home, practice refusing a cigarette, or practice reviewing in your mind the reasons why you don't want to smoke." (*Replacement of undesirable with desirable behavior by mental repetition.*) "Provide yourself with reasonable consequences. Give yourself rewards. Go out to dinner once a week as long as you are sticking to the plan. Perhaps plan a vacation when you have been free of cigarettes for a month." (*Reward for desirable behavior.*) "Think of some simple, fairly immediate, nondestructive punishment. For

When you take something away from a patient, replace it with something else.

Maximize rewards.

example, make yourself do the dishes every evening that you haven't stuck to your plan." (*Negative consequence for undesirable behavior.*)

The more fully the patient understands a problem, its effects on him and his life, its natural history, its treatment, and the consequences of treatment, the greater his sense of control will be. Inversely, his sense of fear and anxiety will decrease. As the patient's sense of control increases and his anxiety decreases, he will be more likely to comply with instructions and actively follow a management plan. The goal of patient education, then, is to give the patient as much understanding of his problem and its management as possible, and as much control of his problem and his destiny as possible. As a result, the patient's attitudes and behaviors relative to his life-style and illness will change.

Try to increase patient autonomy and self-esteem.

COMPLIANCE

The effectiveness of most therapeutic and preventive regimens depends upon patient compliance. Compliance is the degree to which the patient actually molds behaviors and attitudes to fit a therapeutic prescription. Compliance involves keeping appointments; taking medications; following through with advice regarding diet and activity, sleep and stress management, consultations with other clinicians, physiotherapists, and counselors; and embracing the clinician's assessment of the problem and plan for its management.

The patient must *willing* to comply.

The patient must *understand* what he is to do and how his actions affect his health.

Noncompliance is probably the greatest single cause of treatment failure. As mentioned before, compliance cannot be induced or even improved simply with information. Teaching involves transmission of information to the patient so that he understands it. Compliance is not as much affected by the patient's knowledge about his illness or health as it is by the patient's motivation, previous experiences, biases, cultural background, social and environmental factors, and sometimes by the personality effects of the disease process itself.

GOALS

Most practitioners spend about 40% of their direct patient encounter time on patient education. This time is used to inform the patient and enlist his active participation, or to motivate the patient in the management and resolution of his problems. It is important that the patient understand

1. the nature of his problem or diagnosis
2. the problem's underlying causes and its natural history without treatment
3. the expected effects of recommended treatments
4. the range of alternative therapies
5. your plan if the initial therapy is not effective
6. the long-term outlook on his health and life expectancy
7. how to adapt and deal with the problem while it lasts
8. any disability the problem might cause

The patient should understand the purpose of laboratory tests and how the results might affect management. He should understand the signs and symptoms that may develop in the future, and what action he should take in response to them (including reporting them to you). All of the patient's questions and concerns should be addressed openly and clearly. You should learn ways to assess the patient's understanding of what you have told him, ways to resolve misunderstanding and misconceptions, and ways to address latent fears and anxieties.

CRITERIA FOR SUCCESS

As a result of your efforts in patient education, the patient should understand his problem and your instructions adequately enough to follow the instructions appropriately and adhere to the treatment plan. He should be able to take appropriate actions himself in managing, or assisting in managing, his medical problems. Finally, through your efforts, his own efforts, and perhaps with the help of family or other health-care providers, his behavior should change. At subsequent interviews, he will provide you with information about the effects of your therapeutic efforts—both directly through history and physical findings, and indirectly through his behaviors.

Figure 14 summarizes how patient education provides you with additional information to refine your patient problem synthesis, sharpen and confirm your diagnostic impressions, and develop your therapeutic and educational plans. In this way, your patient becomes an active participant in the assessment and understanding of his problems, as well as their management. With the passage of time, particularly in chronic problems such as dia-

Assess your effectiveness in patient education, then modify your plan accordingly.

Patient education and subsequent feedback from the patient become an integral part of your ongoing patient assessment and problem synthesis.

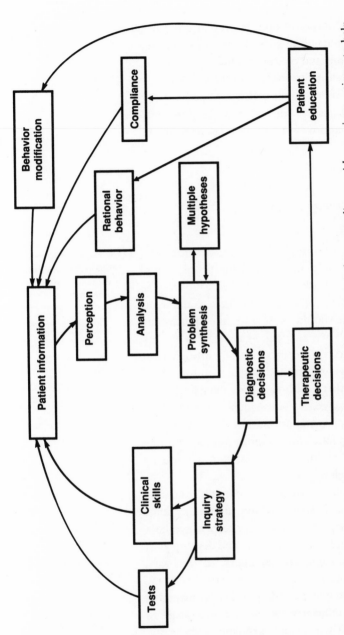

Figure 14. The three primary goals of patient education are to induce compliance with your instructions, to help the patient to gain an understanding sufficient to enable him or her to take rational action, and to change conscious and unconscious behaviors and attitudes through behavior modification. The patient's response to your interventions will modify his or her medical problems and the *patient information* you obtain on subsequent visits, and thus will modify your subsequent problem synthesis and management.

betes, the patient takes more and more responsibility for management, and even for his own continuing education. Your responsibilities decrease as your role becomes more that of advisor and technical specialist. Nothing in practice is more rewarding than following a patient who is gradually assuming effective control of his or her health problems.

PREVENTIVE MEDICINE AND PATIENT EDUCATION

Health, as defined by the World Health Organization conference at Alma Ata, is a state of physical, psychological, and social well-being. The ability to practice wellness requires an understanding of the variables that affect health. These include

1. diet
2. exercise
3. safety in the work place, at home, and on the highway
4. stress management
5. consumption of alcohol, tobacco and other drugs
6. recognition of illness
7. symptomatic treatment of illness
8. management of disabilities (and the maintenance of function in spite of disability)
9. supportive care of family members
10. utilization of health-care services

Although it may not be necessary or appropriate to do so at the initial encounter, you must address all of the patient's health needs and assess his health

Helping the patient minimize health risks and maintain good health through education.

Health is a state of physical, psychological, and social well-being.

You evaluate, manage, and educate the whole person.

risks at some time in your continuing care. Physical, psychological, and social well-being are very closely interrelated. Social, psychological, and physical malaise keep company, and often afflict the same individual. Unfortunately, the existence of social and psychological problems may seriously limit the patient's ability and willingness to participate in patient education or to assume an active, responsible role in management. You must learn to evaluate and to treat the whole person. You must do so with his assistance, but within his limitations.

Medical treatment is a partnership. As you educate the patient, he can gradually assume a greater share of the responsibility and greater autonomy.

Management of a medical problem is a partnership between you and your patient. To work effectively with your patient, you must educate him in the nature of his problem, its natural history, and the nature and effects of therapy. The more your patient understands about the problem and its therapy, the more likely it is that you and he will be able to manage the problem effectively. Education will increase the patient's confidence in you, in the therapeutic plan, and in himself. This increased confidence will be reflected in his attitudes and behaviors and in their effect on the medical problems. Patient education also contributes to your ongoing patient evaluation and problem synthesis (Figure 14).

13

Closing and Documenting the Patient Encounter

The appropriate point for you to close the encounter—how long the encounter should take—depends upon the nature of the patient's problem, its urgency, and the pressures that are on you. Now you must record your findings and decisions in a way that will facilitate your future work with the patient. While you are writing, a little more effort to document your own educational needs relevant to your patient's problems will put you on the road to a lifetime habit of self-education.

CLOSURE, AND THE DURATION OF THE ENCOUNTER

Time adapts to need.

The time taken for a new patient encounter by a clinician is variable. Many clinicians establish a norm for themselves, and usually stick to their concept of how long a patient encounter should take. Primary-care clinicians may use 15-minute

The patient encounter will occupy the time available for it to occur—except in emergencies, when it takes less time.

197

patient encounters. By contrast, some specialists may give themselves an hour. If the patient is felt to represent an emergency, and treatment or tests are urgently needed to forestall serious consequences, the clinician makes the encounter very brief. If the clinician has a busy office with many patients, or if he has an emergency elsewhere, the encounter can be remarkably shortened. By contrast, if the patient has a complex problem, if there is difficulty in communication, if a more extensive examination is needed to find sufficient information to make an appropriate evaluation and treatment decision, or if there is a need for a long conversation with the patient the time of the encounter is often extended.

Some factors will make the encounter longer.

The flexibility of multiple-hypothesis-guided, problem-oriented inquiry strategy allows for both contraction and expansion of the time in the encounter to suit internal or external needs. Under pressure, the clinician quickly develops hypotheses of life-threatening, treatable, or frequent conditions that might explain the patient's presenting problem. The inquiry is incisive, the clinician selecting those questions and examinations that separate hypotheses most effectively and rapidly, spending no time with unnecessary inquiries that would only stall an effective disposition of the patient's problem. You are going to be in this situation many times. This is why you must *practice* your clinical reasoning again and again to be able to perform efficiently and effectively under the pressure of emergencies, or in situations in which time is curtailed. In such circumstances all unnecessary questions are avoided, all unnecessary examinations are avoided, scanning and small talk are sacrificed.

The emergency situation will always test the efficiency and effectiveness of your clinical-reasoning skills.

By contrast, when the problem is difficult, the possible hypotheses are many, and the data acquired do not separate them well, the process can be expanded by the incorporation of a more complete and varied inquiry strategy, the inclusion extra questions and examinations, and the more extensive use of scanning routines.

In the nonurgent situation, by contrast, you have to decide when to quit. Students tend to go on and on asking questions, coming to closure only because the patient or the student is scheduled to go somewhere else or because they are both fatigued. You must decide when further inquiry is no longer productive, and closure is needed. This ability will allow you to suit the length of the encounter to the internal and external pressures around you. The following criteria can be helpful in coming to a decision for closure:

Initially, you must consciously decide when closure is needed.

1. Diagnostic and treatment decisions have been made as well as they are ever going to be at this particular stage of the encounter.
2. Even if good diagnostic decisions or treatment decisions are not possible, no more helpful information is available in this setting at this time.
3. The patient's situation is urgent; tests and treatments are needed.
4. Appropriate treatment has been provided for acute problems, follow-up has been arranged, and appropriate evaluation and management for other problems has been planned and arranged.

DOCUMENTATION: THE
MEDICAL RECORD

Importance of the
medical record.

At closure, you must record a summary of the encounter and your decision. Whether you are in the clinic, office, or inpatient service, there are appropriate forms, sheets, charts, or records for this. The record serves as a reminder of all the facts and decisions you made for your future work with the patient and as a source of communication to others who may become involved in your patient's care. As a communication tool, organization and clarity are of paramount importance. The forms you have to use in a particular clinical setting may ask for a detailed history and physical in a specific format (such as the problem-oriented medical record or a diagnosis-differential diagnosis). Regardless of the format, be certain you have in one way or another recorded the following items:

If the record of your encounter does not tell others—and remind you—of the important data and decisions, the effort expended in your encounter of the patient was in vain. On the other hand, if it rambles on, neither you nor anyone else will read it and try and find the important facts.

1. The presenting picture, or the complaints brought by the patient.
2. The patient's age, sex, occupation, ethnic background, language skills—and your estimate of the patient's reliability in giving a history.
3. Your *problem synthesis*. Remember, this should be a concise, organized description of all the significant data you obtained, free of unnecessary information and free of interpretations of the data. The problem synthesis should stick to the facts and observations (and not include diagnostic labels or interpretations of those facts).

4. Your *diagnostic decisions,* which should be as specific as you consider possible. If you do not have one diagnostic decision, list your alternatives. List any "rule outs" (differential diagnoses). Include psychosocial or situational factors that may be of equal importance in your diagnostic decisions.

5. Your *treatment decisions:* tests, referrals, dispostion of the patient (to home, return visit to the office, admit to the hospital, etc.) follow-up, medications, operations, therapies—whatever.

6. Your *goals of treatment* (your short-term and long-term goals with this particular patient).

7. Any *unresolved matters* that need further attention or that need to be followed as the patient progresses (unresolved symptoms or signs, unresolved laboratory tests, further issues that need to be kept in mind).

These items will document your reasoning process and your decisions, and will not require you or others to read pages and pages of material to be briefed.

THE ENCOUNTER AS A MEANS OF IMPROVING CLINICAL EXPERTISE

Review

Now, on a separate sheet of paper, add the following notes to your copy of the patient's medical record. (You should retain a copy of your patient's record, either printed from your word processor,

Documenting the patient's progress is only half the job—you also must document your clinical performance.

photocopied, or—if necessary—rewritten, as this copy is important for your files and for your own personal learning).

1. The length of time you took in the patient encounter.

2. The hypotheses you generated at the *very beginning* of the encounter. Try to be as honest in your recollection as possible (refer to your note pad).

3. Your assessment of your own ability in working with the patient, using whatever comments seem appropriate. In doing this, review your ability and comfort in the following areas:

   a. initial concept formulation (defining the patient's problem)
   b. hypothesis generation
   c. inquiry strategy design
   d. clinical skills performance
   e. problem synthesis (data base)
   f. assembling a logical pathophysiologic mechanism for the patient's picture
   g. diagnostic decision-making
   h. therapeutic decision-making
   i. determination of closure
   j. record-keeping ability

4. The items of clinical or basic science information you wish you knew, or at least knew better, in working with this patient to effectively carry out (a) through (j) above. This includes unanswered questions raised by the encounter. This list could include answers to the following:

   a. What are the appropriate hypotheses for the problem presented by the patient?

b. What knowledge is needed about the frequency of symptoms, signs, or the course of certain diseases or conditions?

c. What are the possible underlying pathophysiologic mechanisms or anatomic, physiologic, or biochemical abnormalities that could be responsible for the symptoms, signs, or laboratory results seen?

d. Are there alternate techniques and physical examination appropriate to the problem?

e. Are there more appropriate laboratory or diagnostic tests to resolve the hypotheses entertained?

f. Can the sensitivity, specificity, risks, morbidity, or mortality of certain procedures be established or estimated?

g. What other medications might be considered? (Include a consideration of their actions, pharmacokinetics, reactions with other drugs, contraindications, and side effects.)

h. Are there more appropriate treatment or management procedures available?

And many more—*think carefully.*

Review your encounter carefully. In addition to those listed above, ask yourself the following kinds of questions (and write down any significant answers).

- Did you recognize the problem well enough to pull together an initial concept?
- Did you understand the symptoms and signs that were presented?
- Were you able to come up with reasonable initial hypotheses?

Self-assessment, the way to self-directed learning.

- Did you have sufficient information about those hypotheses to inquire against them?
- Did you know good laboratory or diagnostic tests to separate the hypotheses?
- Did you order redundant or unnecessary tests?
- Could you decide whether the patient's problems matched your hypotheses?
- Did you know which tests and treatment to employ?
- Did you know what results to expect if your hypothesis was correct?
- Of those tests you did consider, were you comfortable with your knowledge of their benefit/cost aspects? Could you decide on closure?
- If the problem was urgent, was your inquiry focused, efficient, and effective?
- Was your treatment based on a knowledge of the probable course of the suspected illness in this patient and did it consider all the benefit/cost aspects?

March yourself through the encounter, and challenge your thinking in this manner. Note down what you need to learn, or learn better, and which questions you need to answer to work more effectively if this kind of patient problem should occur again. Undertake this review *right after* the patient encounter—not a moment later—while the whole encounter is fresh in your mind. This document is your *ticket* to becoming an expert clinician.

As you continue this review process after every patient encounter, you will get better and better at self-assessment, and you will become more aware of your own performance and your educational needs. This self-monitoring and self-assessment should become a well-performed lifetime habit.

While you are building basic skills, you should learn to dictate the record of the encounter, if that is possible. Dictation is a difficult, but time-saving, skill that is learned only by practice—start early. The result will not only be less time and effort, but it can produce an easier-to-read document. If you really want to move into the contemporary world, use computer software to organize and record your patient information.

Learn to dictate your patient records, and move into computer-processed records, as soon as you are able.

Follow-Up

In this book we have concentrated on your initial encounter with the patient. In most instances you will need to follow your patient over time to complete your diagnostic decisions, initiate appropriate treatment, and follow the result of treatment or the course of the patient. The location of the next encounter could be your office, a clinic, or the hospital. Wherever the encounter occurs, it essentially duplicates the process described so far in this book. In most instances it will be in a markedly abbreviated form. Often you will have received test results, which you will analyze for significant facts to add to your problem synthesis—possibly resulting in a change to your working hypothesis or diagnosis.

On the follow-up visit you will interview and examine the patient to uncover any changes in symptoms and signs, new findings, or evidence of improvement or worsening, and to undertake a review of the patient's problem for more facts

Your diagnosis at the end of the encounter was a working hypothesis, to be improved and modified by subsequent experience with the patient. Your treatment decisions must be followed for your patient's benefit and your own education.

that may be added to the problem synthesis in light of your diagnostic decisions. It is always the same process: you start with a patient and any additional records, then carry on your clinical-reasoning process to evaluate your previous hypothesis (or hypotheses) and make appropriate evaluative and treatment decisions.

14

Continuing Medical Education for the Clinician

In this chapter you are introduced to the powerful educational effectiveness of problem-based, self-directed learning. The process employs well-established principles of educational psychology to move you more effectively into medical expertise and to help you develop a lifetime pattern of learning through self-directed study.

THE PATH TO SELF-IMPROVEMENT AND LIFE-LONG LEARNING

As mentioned in the preceding chapter, your written notes regarding your performance in the patient encounter can be your ticket to acquiring expert clinical-reasoning skills. There are several important stages to carrying out your own continued medical education.

Self-Monitoring

The ability to continuously reflect on your own thinking and progress, to reflect upon and review your thoughts and decisions during a patient encounter, is critical to self-improvement. You must practice being deliberately aware of what you are thinking, and why, until it becomes a habit. There is no room for impulsive thinking in medicine (not to be confused with the rapid, seemingly unconsious, decision-making of the expert clinician described in the first chapters).

Self-Assessment

Self-assessment was described in the last chapter. In brief, it requires an ability to sense where your knowledge and skills may not be sufficient (self-assessment occurs during the monitoring process).

Defining Learning Needs

Write down the subjects that need study, the questions that need answers, the topics to be reviewed, and the new skills to be acquired.

Identifying Learning Resources

What would be the best, most accurate, most feasible or practical resources to use to satisfy your learning needs? You must gain experience in finding effective and efficient ways to get appropriate facts and answers in particular learning areas. In the beginning, this is a process of trial and error.

There are many informational resources at hand. It would probably be wise to concentrate on those kinds of resources that will always be available to you no matter where you go in your future practice. Such resources are textbooks, journals, monographs, yearbook reviews, specialists in various medical disciplines, other health professionals, and a variety of computer searches (now available in most libraries probably to come in many other settings, such as hospitals or offices). You must bear in mind that textbooks can treat subjects superficially and often do not contain exceptions to classical entities. However, they do have the advantage of surveying a broad area. However, always look at a textbook's copyright date (and realize that the newest information in a new textbook is, at best, a year old by the time you read it). Reviews appearing in monographs that are published within a year or two of your search may contain more contemporary information. Journal articles provide even more up-to-date information and in considerably greater depth.

Finding the right information source quickly and easily is an essential skill that comes only from practice.

Lastly, the most up-to-date information occurs in conferences or meetings in your field. When you read medical literature or talk to experts, consultants, or colleagues, be sure to consider the accuracy and reliability of the data you are receiving. This is particularly true of research reports, especially clinical trials; you must be able to critique the methods used and the results obtained.

Using Learning Resources

You should know how to use all resources appropriately. Refer to *Index Medicus, MESH, Excerpta Medica, Current Contents,* and *Science*

Citation Index to find appropriate information sources as mentioned above. Computerized information resources in a variety of subjects are becoming more and more plentiful, and more easily accessed. A librarian can always assist you in these matters. Computer searches for a particular subject may be one of the more efficient ways of obtaining reasonably up-to-date and highly relevant information to meet your learning needs. You should become adept at using these resources. They are very useful, and will eventually represent an accepted standard for obtaining timely information about diagnosis and new therapies, as well as information about new complications with accepted therapies. Never overlook the value of an expert in the particular area about which you are concerned. A conversation with an expert can save you a lot of time by providing you with the quick answers you need and referring you to resources you can subsequently study. An expert is always aware of contemporary writings in his or her field. However, even with an expert, it is wise to ask for data references and to double-check them yourself.

Coping With Frustrations

Self-assessment and self-directed learning—the skills of life-long continuing education.

When you begin to undertake self-education, you will become frustrated for one of two reasons. Oftentimes you will spend a great deal of time to find and study a resource only to discover that it does not really give you the information you needed. Other times you will find resources that give you an inappropriate level of information: some sources will give you far more information in greater detail than you require, others will be superficial. As with anything else, in research and study practice makes perfect. *The earlier you jump in the water and start to swim, the better off you will be.* In a short period of time, you will develop efficient and effective self-educational skills that will help you immeasurably, not only in your clinical care of patients but also in your learning within medical school.

As you study disease entities, do not try to memorize the demographic details, symptoms, signs, and disease courses. Be sure you understand the pathophysiology of the disease, why it strikes the people of the age and sex it does, and why it produces the clinical phenomenology seen in patients. Then reconstruct all the details from this underlying story whenever you need them. This basic-science story will help you to recall this disease in future work and to deduce its possible presence through inquiry.

You should also start now with a personal filing system to return to any resource when you need it again. Your librarian can help you set one up, either in file-card form or on a personal computer.

Applying Clinical Knowledge

When you have studied to better understand a patient you have just encountered, go back again to the documents you have written concerning the patient problem (described in the previous chapter). Take a red pen and go over your records in a careful sequence. Now that study has made you an expert about the patient problem, write down in the appropriate places on those documents the following data:

Now that study has made you expert, *use* the information immediately or the value of your study will not be fully realized.

1. Information or observations you should have noticed when you first encountered the patient.

2. Changes you should have made in your initial hypotheses (hypotheses you should have included, hypotheses you should not have included, hypotheses that could have been stated more clearly, etc.).

3. Areas where the problem synthesis was lacking or uninformative. In noting this, you may also need to note down the kinds of inquiries that you should have made in working up the patient to better separate the hypotheses you entertained, or the new hypotheses you now think you should have been entertained (item 2 above), and the kinds of information that should be included in your problem synthesis.

4. Changes you should make in your diagnostic decision.

5. Changes you should make in your technique of assessment or your use of your clinical-reasoning skills with this particular patient problem, (and future problems similar to this one).

   Once this critique has been completed and you have had an opportunity to reflect on what you have learned, write down on your second document a brief summary of what this patient experience has taught you and the implications for subsequent patients of what you have learned.

   If you have the opportunity to follow the patient or to see the patient again, apply what you have learned to the patient's care.

   As you follow the patient, record the results

of the tests that have been ordered, the patient's response to treatment (including the autopsy result if the patient dies). Feed this information back into your records. You will eventually need to keep files of your patient records, either in a cabinet or a computer. These files will become an extremely valuable record for you, and will enhance your evolving clinical memory.

It cannot be stressed enough how much you will learn with this approach. Although it may seem to require a lot of extra work over and above your regular tasks, it will become easy and automatic once you get used to it. You must get used to this cycle:

1. documentation
2. self-evaluation
3. self-education
4. reapplication of new learning to the patient problem
5. summarization of what has been learned

Do this until it has become habit. You will soon realize that it provides one of the most effective learning experiences possible. Great strides will be made both in your clinical-reasoning skills (your scientific approach to your patient) and in your usable knowledge base.

Using Time Constrictions to Obtain Confidence in Your Professional Skill

One last maneuver is necessary to put the final professional touches on your clinical-reasoning skills, to ensure that you will have reflexly effective,

Moving into the professional arena with skill and confidence by practice under pressure.

efficient skills at your command, to be performed almost without thinking. You never know when you are going to run into an urgent patient situation that will require you to apply your skills comfortably, efficiently, and effectively in a crisis. Therefore, if in your last patient encounter you took an hour to take a history, do a physical examination, educate the patient, and provide a management plan *then lay down the law* and discipline yourself to take only 50 minutes at the next encounter. At the end your performance in problem synthesis and decision-making should be as good as when you took an hour. Once fifty minutes is comfortable, then cut off more time until you can work effectively in half an hour or less.

You will find this time-cutting very uncomfortable and you will initially be unwilling to do it, because there always will be more information you feel you should get. However, it is the way to develop effective professional skills. You will learn to cut down on unnecessary questions and examinations. Find every opportunity to work with patient problems and force yourself to take progressively less time with each new patient, putting on the pressure. This is not unlike the way a musician must practice to become an accomplished performer on an instrument, or how an athlete must practice to achieve professional ability. There will always be exceptions, certain patient problems where more time is necessary to deal adequately with the problems presented. However, if you are efficient where possible, then you will feel even more relaxed and comfortable when that confused, uncooperative patient with a complex, emotional, difficult problem walks in and requires much of your time and understanding.

Force yourself to have not only an accurate, but also an efficient, reasoning process. Time constrictions force your generation of hypotheses to be quick and effective, your inquiry search to contain only those actions that will produce significant information, and your scanning to be crisp. *You cannot afford to wander down wrong paths.* By disciplining yourself now you will achieve a final reward, a feeling of confidence in your clinical skills, and enjoyment in your ability to work with all kinds of patient problems in almost any circumstance.

CONCLUDING PEARLS

It is the authors' hope that you will practice scientific clinical reasoning skills at every opportunity.

- To develop an accurate initial concept, look carefully for important initial information as the patient encounter begins.
- Generate a complete set of hypotheses in every patient encounter, carefully watching their degree of specificity and their complimentarity. Be sure to watch out for hidden biases.
- Use your creativity, and your inductive skills, to develop these hypotheses.
- Use your critical deductive skills to inquire in a manner that will establish the more likely hypothesis.
- Generate new hypotheses whenever your inquiry becomes unproductive or new data makes your present hypotheses less likely.

- Carefully assemble a problem synthesis from the significant data obtained from your hypothesis-guided inquiry.
- Employ consistent and accurate clinical skills.
- In both your hypotheses-generation and inquiry strategy, be guided by an awareness of the basic pathophysiologic mechanisms that may be operative in your patient's problem.
- Think of past patient experiences similar to the one you are facing now, and what was productive or unproductive about them.
- Force yourself to make diagnostic and therapeutic decisions even in situations where there is ambiguity or lack of important information.
- In your choice of subsequent tests and a management plan, be aware of benefit/cost factors.
- Consider carefully the educational needs of your patient and employ the appropriate educational strategy.
- As you work with your patient, constantly ask yourself if you have all the facts or skills you need to evaluate and care for your patient and to keep yourself contemporary with medical knowledge.
- Note the areas you need to study, and go to appropriate resources to gain the information and skills you need.
- Apply newly acquired knowledge and skills to the problem, and note how you would have handled the problem differently after review.

Do these things the rest of your professional life. You will become an expert clinician, and the profession of medicine will be an exciting and rewarding career for you. Good luck!

Selected References

THE CLINICAL-REASONING PROCESS

Barrows HS, Bennett K. Experimental studies on the diagnostic (problem-solving) skill of the neurologist, their implications for neurological training. *Arch Neurol.* 1972;26(3):273–277.

Barrows HS, Norman GR, Neufeld VR, Feightner JW. The clinical reasoning of randomly selected physicians in general medical practice. *Clin Invest Med.* 1982;5(1):49–55.

Barrows HS, Tamblyn RM. *Problem-Based Learning: An Approach to Medical Education.* New York, N.Y.: Springer; 1980.

Eddy DM, Clayton CH. The art of diagnosis: solving the clinicopathological exercise. *N Engl J Med.* 1982;306:1263–1268.

Elstein AS, Shulman LS, Sprafka SS. *An Analysis of Medical Inquiry Process.* Cambridge, Mass.: Harvard University Press; 1978.

Glaser R. Education and thinking. *Am Psychol.* 1984;39(1):93–104.

Schon DA. *The Reflective Practitioner.* New York: Basic Books; 1983.

THE CONTENT ASPECT OF CLINICAL PERFORMANCE

These references concentrate on the knowledge clinicians must have about diseases and symptoms and how they should be approached (see discussion in Chapter 1).

Beck P, Byyny RL, Adams KS. *Case Exercises in Clinical Reasoning.* Chicago, Ill: Year Book Medical Publishers; 1981.

Cutler P. *Problem Solving in Clinical Medicine: From Data to Diagnosis.* 2nd ed. Baltimore, Md.: Williams & Wilkins; 1985.

Dijkhuis HJPM, Izenberg N, Kooy SVD. *Problem Solving in Primary Medical Care: Its Procedure, Evaluation, and Teaching. An Introduction with Case Histories.* Leiden, Neth.: Apruyt, Van Mantgem & DeBoew, BV; 1986.

Fraser RC. *Clinical Method: A General Practice Approach.* London: Butterworths; 1987.

Fulginiti VA. *Pediatric Clinical Problem Solving.* Baltimore, Md.: Williams & Wilkins; 1981.

Heilman KM, Watson RT, Greer M. *Handbook for Differential Diagnosis of Neurological Signs and Symptoms.* 2nd ed. London: Butterworths; 1988.

Hurst JW. *Medicine for the Practicing Physician.* 2nd ed. Boston/London: Butterworths; 1988.

Sheldon SH, Levy HB. *Pediatric Differential Diagnosis: A Problem-Oriented Approach.* New York, N.Y.: Raven; 1985.

CLINICAL DECISION-MAKING

These are books and journal articles that discuss the decision-making process. They describe the probabilistic approaches to making decisions about diagnosis, laboratory and diagnostic investigations, and treatment.

Anderson RE, Hill RB, Key C. The sensitivity and specificity of clinical diagnostics during five decades: towards an understanding of necessary fallibility. *JAMA*. 1989; 261(11):1610–1617.

Balla JI. *The Diagnostic Process: A Model for Clinical Teachers*. Cambridge, Eng.: Cambridge University Press; 1985.

Balla JI. Logical thinking in the diagnostic process. *Methods Inf Med*. 1980;19(2):88–92.

Murphy EA. *The Logic of Medicine*. Baltimore, Md.: Johns Hopkins University Press; 1976.

Pauker SG, Kassirer JP. Decision analysis (medical progress). *N Engl J Med*. 1987;316(5):250–258.

Sackett DL, Haynes RB, Tugwell P. *Clinical Epidemiology*. Boston/Toronto: Little, Brown & Company; 1985.

Sox HC Jr. *Medical Decision Making*. London: Butterworths; 1988.

Weinstein MC, Fineberg HV. *Clinical Decision Analysis*. Philadelphia, Penn.: WB Saunders; 1980.

PATIENT EDUCATION

Donaldson MC, London CD. Time study of doctors and nurses at two Swedish health care centers: Swedish Health Center Doctors and Nurses. *Med Care*. 1971;9:457.

Haynes RB, et al., eds. *Compliance in Health Care*. Baltimore, Md.: Johns Hopkins University Press; 1979.

Hessle SJ, Haggerty RJ. General pediatrics: A study of practice in the mid-1960's. *J Pediatr*. 1968;73:271.

Levine DM, et al. Health education for hypertensive patients. *JAMA*. 1979;241:1700.

Miller L, Goldstein J. More efficient care of diabetic patients in a country hospital setting. *N Engl J Med*. 1972;286:1388.

Morisky DE, et al. Five-year blood pressure control and mortality following health education for hypertensive patients. *Am J Public Health*. In press.

Rakel RE. *Textbook of Family Practice*, 3rd ed. Philadelphia, Penn.: WB Saunders Co.; 1984.

Skinner BF, Vaughan ME. *Enjoy Old Age: Living Fully in Your Later Years*. New York, N.Y.: Warner Books; 1983.

Society of Teachers of Family Medicine, National Task Force on Training Family Physicians in Patient Education. *Patient Education: A Handbook for Teachers*. Kansas City, Kan.: 1979.

Watson DL, Tharp RG. *Self-Directed Behavior: Self-Modification for Personal Adjustment*. Monterey, Calif.: Brooks/Cole Publishing Co.; 1977.

World Health Organization. Declaration of Alma-Ata. World Health Organization Conference at Alma-Ata, Kazakstan, Soviet Republic, 9/1978. *Lancet*. 1978;2(8098):1040–1041.

INFORMATICS

These resources provide a background for the rapidly evolving field of informatics. Soon practicing physicians will incorporate the infinite powers of memory, computation, and information retrieval of the computer into their own ongoing reasoning processes as they are working with their patient problems.

Barnett GO, Cimino JG, Hupp JA, Hoffer EP. DXLplain: An evolving diagnostic decision-support system, *JAMA*. 1987;258(1):67–74.

Haynes RB, Ramsden M, McKibbon KA, Walker CJ, Ryan NC. A review of medical education and medical informatics. *Acad Med*. 1989; 207–212.

Shortliffe EH. Computer Programs to Support Clinical Decision Making. *JAMA*. 1987;258(1):61–66.

PROBLEM SIMULATIONS

These are printed resources for clinical problems that can be used for practice and learning clinical-reasoning skills.

Problem-Based Learning Modules (PBLM). A series of patient problems that can be interviewed and examined with the same freedom as occurs in the real clinical situation. They also serve as resource for problem-based learning. Contact Linda Distlehorst, Southern Illinois University School of Medicine, P.O. Box 19230, Springfield, Illinois 62794–9230.

Waterman RE, Duban SL, Mennin SP, Kaufman A. *Clinical Problem-Based Learning: A Workbook for Integrating Basic and Clinical Science*. Albuquerque, N.M.: University of New Mexico Press; 1988.

Index